D0639407

Clinical Handbook for Kozier & Erb's Fundamentals of Nursing

Concepts, Process, and Practice

NINTH EDITION

Berman • Snyder

PEARSON

Boston Columbus Indianapolis New York San Francisco Upper Saddle River
Amsterdam Cape Town Dubai London Madrid Milan Munich Paris Montreal Toronto
Delhi Mexico City São Paulo Sydney Hong Kong Seoul Singapore Taipei Tokyo

Library of Congress Cataloging-in-Publication Data
Berman, Audrey.
Clinical handbook for Kozier & Erb's fundamentals of nursing: concepts, process, and practice / Berman, Snyder. — 9th ed.
p. ; cm.
Includes index.
ISBN-13: 978-0-13-802464-2
ISBN-10: 0-13-802464-2
1. Nursing—Handbooks, manuals, etc. I. Snyder, Shirlee. II. Kozier & Erb's fundamentals of nursing. 9th ed. III. Title.
[DNLM: 1. Nursing Process—Handbooks. 2. Nursing Care—Handbooks. 3. Nursing Theory—Handbooks. WY 49]
RT41.F8813 2011
610.73—dc22
2011012480

Notice: Care has been taken to confirm the accuracy of information presented in this book. The authors, editors, and the publisher, however, cannot accept any responsibility for errors or omissions or for consequences from application of the information in this book and make no warranty, express or implied, with respect to its contents. The authors and publisher have exerted every effort to ensure that drug selections and dosages set forth in this text are in accord with current recommendations and practice at time of publication. However, in view of ongoing research, changes in government regulations, and the constant flow of information relating to drug therapy and drug reactions, the reader is urged to check the package inserts of all drugs for any change in indications of dosage and for added warnings and precautions. This is particularly important when the recommended agent is a new and/or infrequently employed drug.

Copyright © 2012, 2008, 2004 by Pearson Education, Inc., Upper Saddle River, New Jersey 07458. Pearson Prentice Hall. All rights reserved. Printed in the United States of America. This publication is protected by Copyright and permission should be obtained from the publisher prior to any prohibited reproduction, storage in a retrieval system, or transmission in any form or by any means, electronic, mechanical, photocopying, recording, or likewise. For information regarding permission(s), write to: Rights and Permissions Department.

Pearson® is a registered trademark of Pearson plc

PEARSON

www.pearsonhighered.com

10 9 8 7 6 5 4 3 2 1
ISBN-10: 0-13-802464-2
ISBN-13: 978-0-13-802464-2

Contents

Preface vi

Introduction vii

Reviewers xv

Unit 1 Fundamental Nursing

A. Components of the Nursing Process 2

B. Aspects of Delegation 4

C. Communication Guidelines 7

1. SBAR Communication Guidelines 15
2. Handoff Communication/Change-of-Shift Report 17
3. Telephone and Verbal Orders 19

Unit 2 Assessment and Diagnosis

A. Nursing Health History 22

B. Methods of Examining 28

C. Vital Signs 30

D. Physical Health Examination 36

E. Nursing Diagnoses 61

Unit 3 Planning and Implementation

A. Safety Guidelines 70

1. Guidelines Related to Body Mechanics and Safe Client Handling and Movement 71
2. Preventing Falls in Health Care Agencies 73
3. Adult Home Hazard Appraisal 74
4. Steps to Follow in the Event of Fire 75

B. Clinical Guidelines 77

1. Fluid and Electrolyte Balance 77
2. Individualizing Care for Clients with Pain 83
3. Respiratory Function 87
4. Tube Feedings 91
5. Urinary Elimination 96
6. Fecal Elimination 100
7. Pressure Areas 103
8. Healing Wounds 114
9. Postoperative Period 116

C. Teaching and Learning Guidelines 119

D. Medications 125

1. Methods of Calculating Dosages 129
2. Injection Techniques 135

Unit 4 Documentation and Evaluation

A. Documentation 144

1. Ethical and Legal Considerations 144
2. Ensuring Confidentiality of Computer Records 144
3. Charting Guidelines 145
4. Essential Client Information 146

B. Documentation Formats 148
1. Narrative 148
2. SOAP 149
3. Focus Charting (DAR) 149
C. Evaluation 153

Unit 5 Quick Reference

A. Standard Precautions and Infection Control Strategies 156
B. Common Abbreviations and "Do Not Use" Abbreviations 164
C. Medical Terminology: Root Words, Prefixes, and Suffixes 168
D. Weight and Volume Conversions and Equivalents 176
E. Laboratory Values 178
F. Common Diagnostic Studies 197
G. Nursing Interventions for Endoscopic Examinations 199
H. Studies of The Gastrointestinal Tract 203
I. Studies of The Gallbladder and Bile Ducts 205
J. Radiographic Studies: Intravenous Pyelography, Angiography, Myelography 208
K. Key Information About Vitamins 211
L. Key Information About Minerals 215
M. Key Information About Trace Minerals 217

Glossary 221

Index 249

PREFACE

The *Clinical Handbook for Kozier & Erb's Fundamentals of Nursing*, 9e serves as a resource for students in the clinical area. It provides succinct information to guide you as you begin this important, exciting, and challenging component of your nursing program.

To keep this practical guide compact and portable, we have summarized key information designed to reinforce content that first must be learned thoroughly and carefully from *Fundamentals of Nursing*. The *Clinical Handbook* is not intended in any way to replace the text; rather, its purpose is to help you recall key points as you prepare to deliver safe and effective nursing care in a dynamic clinical environment. Before proceeding with the suggested guidelines and actions given in this book, check to determine an agency's policies, practices, and protocols.

The *Clinical Handbook* opens with a fundamental nursing unit that introduces the nursing process, delegation principles, and communication guidelines. Unit 2 reviews the processes for conducting a health history and physical examination. A complete list of the current North American Nursing Diagnosis Association (NANDA) nursing diagnoses is included. In Unit 3, we provide summaries of clinically related topics that you can expect to encounter routinely. Unit 4 presents documentation and evaluation principles. The handbook ends with a quick reference unit that presents essential information you will be able to retrieve rapidly. As you gain expertise in the clinical area, we believe you will continue to consult the *Clinical Handbook* again and again.

Introduction

On the first day of my pediatrics rotation, one of the children assigned to me was a 6-year-old asthmatic previously hospitalized several times for this same problem. Walking into his room with my instructor, I put forth what I thought was an air of confidence, even though my heart was beating a mile a minute. After the introductions, my little client reached for my hand and, with a voice of authority, told me not to be nervous, because he would tell me what I was supposed to do. Even though I was a little embarrassed that my cover was blown by a 6-year-old, I had to chuckle at being comforted by the client I was supposed to make comfortable. Welcome to the world of clinical rotations!

Clinical experiences give the student the opportunity to translate classroom theory and laboratory skills into action. This necessary and exciting part of nursing education, however, is often accompanied by feelings of apprehension and awkwardness. New situations heighten these feelings, as does the realization that you are still in transition between learning a skill and knowing how to use it efficiently. However, by being organized, being an active learner, and being good to yourself, you can use these feelings to challenge yourself and turn your clinical experiences into fun learning experiences.

Nursing is undergoing a wonderful evolution, and as a student, you bring fresh views to the process. The clients you will care for, the staff you will work with, and the facts you will learn about yourself will help shape your views and turn you into the competent professional you want to be. No matter how difficult your day is, you should look on it as a learning experience. These difficult days give you precious knowledge that will make future days go easier. The following are tips to help you avoid some of the pitfalls that make the clinical experience unnecessarily stressful.

ORGANIZE

Clinical days always bring a little apprehension. Even when the routines were familiar and the knowledge base was more solid, I still asked myself: "What will my instructor ask me? What emergencies will upset the schedule I set for myself? What if I oversleep and I'm late?"

To help combat this apprehension, I always reminded myself that there was nothing routine about client care, even though people talked about "hospital routines." There are only two predictable actions in nursing: (1) Clients will be cared for, and (2) documentation must be done. Everything else is subject to change!

To maintain your cool, do your work efficiently, and feel satisfied at the end of the day, you must be organized, set priorities, and remain flexible. Even if nothing else in your life is organized, be organized in your approach to the clinical experience. Remember also that organization and the ability to set priorities are behaviors instructors look for and grade on. The following are suggestions to help you become better organized:

- Arrive early. Set your alarm clock so that you arrive at the clinical site at least 20 minutes early. This gives you time to review the charts for any changes in orders, any orders that may have expired, or anything that requires your client to leave the nursing unit. Doing this applies even if you cared for the same client the day before. Building in extra time also helps you on days when traffic is heavy or when you hit the snooze button once too often. The clinical experience can be stressful, so manage the stressors that are self-induced.
- Make a worksheet for reviewing charts. Without violating privacy rules, include the initials of the

client, room number, diagnosis, primary nurse, times to assess vital signs, times to administer medications, equipment needs, procedures, and a space for comments. By making a note of the equipment you need, you can minimize the number of trips to the supply room (e.g., for dressing changes). Write in red all procedures or medications that are time sensitive. In addition to helping you organize your information, this also facilitates note writing and reporting to the primary nurse. See page xii for a blank sample worksheet you can use.

- If possible, check the client's medications when you get to the nursing unit. In some cases, medications are stored in secured cabinets, and students may not be permitted independent access to the keys or electronic codes. One of the most stressful situations you can face is to find yourself running late because of an intervening emergency, only to discover that the client's medications are not on the unit; meanwhile, your instructor is waiting for you to give the medications. By checking the Medication Administration Record, you can prepare yourself for this situation. If an order has expired, notify the primary nurse promptly.
- Attend report and/or talk to the primary nurse before you start. As a student, you must act as independently as possible in assessments and decision making; however, the primary nurse has ultimate responsibility for the client's care. In particular, find out about special circumstances relating to the client. For example, the primary nurse may tell you that the client does not eat breakfast until his wife arrives at 8:30 A.M. If this is not written in the chart, you may get yourself into a conflict with the client and learn about his preference the hard way. Knowing the details ahead of time can make your day easier.
- Do an "eyeball assessment" of each client's room before you start your day. Introduce yourself to the client and ensure that the client is safe and does not require

Client's Initials/Rm # Diagnosis Primary RN	Vital Signs Blood Sugars	Medication Times	IVs Catheters I & O	Treatments Procedures	Comments

any immediate care. Then look at whatever equipment is in the room. (Do not perform a detailed examination of the client; you will do that when your shift begins.) Is there an IV? Is it dated and timed? Is it about to run out? Is there a catheter? Is the client being tube-fed? You will go over this information in the report, but having it beforehand can help make you a more active participant.

On your first day in a new nursing unit or hospital, you will receive an orientation to the unit. After this orientation, do your own inspection and find out how the supply room is organized—for example, where the 4 × 4 gauzes, catheter setups, and so on, are located. Review fire exits and where emergency equipment such as the "code" cart and fire extinguishers are located. Also, find out where the staff bathroom is! When you get busy, it is nice to be able to save steps.

By staying organized and taking control of those things that you can, you can minimize stress and develop good habits that will stay with you throughout your career.

SETTING PRIORITIES

Priority setting is the process of establishing a preferential sequence for addressing nursing diagnoses and interventions. The nurse and client begin planning by deciding which nursing diagnosis requires attention first. Instead of rank-ordering diagnoses, nurses can group them as having high, medium, or low priority. Life-threatening problems are high priority. Health-threatening problems are assigned medium priority. A low-priority problem is one that arises from normal developmental needs or that requires only minimal nursing support.

Nurses frequently use Maslow's hierarchy of needs when setting priorities. Physiological needs such as air, food, and water are basic to life and receive higher priority than the need for security or activity. Growth needs, such as self-esteem, are not perceived as "basic" in this framework.

It is not necessary to resolve all high-priority diagnoses before addressing others. The nurse may partially address a high-priority diagnosis and then deal with a diagnosis of lesser priority. Furthermore, because the client may have several problems, the nurse often deals with more than one diagnosis at a time.

Priorities change as the client's responses, problems, and therapies change. The nurse must consider a variety of factors when assigning priorities, including the following:

1. Client's health values and beliefs. Values concerning health may be more important to the nurse than to the client. When there is such a difference of opinion, the client and nurse should discuss it openly to resolve any conflict.
2. Client's priorities. Involving the client in prioritizing and care planning enhances cooperation. Sometimes, however, the client's perception of what is important conflicts with the nurse's knowledge of potential problems or complications.
3. Resources available to the nurse and client. If finances, equipment, or personnel are scarce in a health care agency, then a problem may be given a lower priority than usual.
4. Urgency of the health problem. Regardless of the framework used, life-threatening situations require that the nurse assign them high priority. Situations that affect the integrity of the client, that is, those that could have a negative or destructive effect on the client, also have high priority.
5. Medical treatment plan. The priorities for treating health problems must be congruent with treatment by other health professionals.

LEARN BEYOND THE HERE AND NOW

Nursing practice is based on understanding how to integrate knowledge from many sources and how to translate theory and facts into action. Clinical experiences offer a wonderful opportunity to do this, but keep in mind that you need to focus primarily on how to help the client. Sometimes, the pressure to perform well for a good grade gets in the way of the learning experience. However, if you focus on the needs of your client, a good grade will follow. As a nursing student, you have many ways to learn about nursing while still placing highest priority on your client's needs. Review all pathophysiology and nursing theory related to your client's diagnosis, no matter how confident you feel about your knowledge base. After reviewing the pathophysiology, jot down the laboratory studies, procedures, and medications you would expect to find ordered on the chart.

Also jot down signs and symptoms you would expect to see in the client and potential complications. Compare your list to what actually appears in the chart. Compare your assessment findings with what you put on your list. How do the lists differ? How are they the same? Do not let your title, "nursing student," prevent you from being an active member of the health care team.

Ask questions of and talk with your instructor, other nurses, and other members of the health care team. Remember, the only dumb question is the one not asked. Read journal articles that relate to your clients' diagnoses.

After you leave the unit, make it a point to look for a new journal article that pertains to at least one of your clients. Imagine the pleasure of being able to answer an instructor's question about a client's course of treatment with, "A study reported in the latest issue of *Nursing Research* found that. . . ." This not only makes a positive impression, but also helps you learn. Although it may be tough to fit into your schedule, reading journals should become a habit.

TAKE CARE OF YOURSELF

Above all else, take care of yourself. There is no way to give good client care if you cannot concentrate because you are hungry or frazzled.

- Eat a good meal before clinical rotations. It may sound trite, but given the unpredictability of the hospital day, you cannot always depend on having time for a break.
- Organize your things the day before.

- If you drive, make sure the car has gas. There is nothing worse than realizing that your tank is empty, and all the gas stations are closed.
- Keep some raisins or your favorite energy booster in your pocket for a quick pickup.
- If you are feeling harried, stop for a minute, and take a deep breath or two.
- Do not ever be afraid to ask for help.
- Keep a sense of humor.

Like anything else, the process of learning nursing can be frightening at first. The idea of practicing on real clients can be worrisome. However, with some thinking beforehand and assertiveness, you can make the process fun, challenging, and a source of wonderful stories to tell for years to come.

Best wishes for a great career in nursing.

Merilyn D. Francis, BSN, RN
1994 Graduate, University of the District of Columbia
(edited 2011)

Reviewers

We would like to sincerely thank our student and faculty reviewers for their thoughtful feedback and suggestions.

Gerri DiBartolo
Nevada State College
Henderson, NV

Kelly Mecham, RN, MSN, FNP-BC
Nevada State College
Henderson, NV

Linda L. Robertson, PhD, RN
La Roche College
Pittsburgh, PA

Sandra Lea, Ed.D., RN
Baptist College of Health Sciences
Memphis, TN

Talitha Canaan, CRNA, MSN
Samuel Merritt University
Sacramento, CA

UNIT 1

FUNDAMENTAL NURSING

A. Components of the Nursing Process
B. Aspects of Delegation
C. Communication Guidelines
   1. SBAR Communication Guidelines
   2. Handoff Communication/ Change-of-Shift Report
   3. Telephone and Verbal Orders

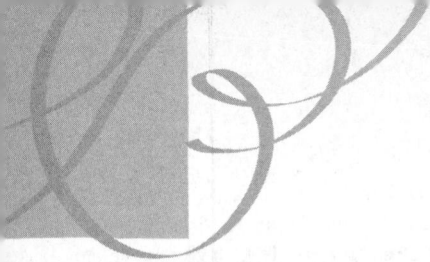

A. Components of the Nursing Process

The nursing process is a systematic, rational method of planning and providing individualized nursing care. Its goal is to identify a client's health status and actual or potential health care problems, to establish plans to meet the identified needs, and to deliver specific nursing interventions to meet those needs. The nursing process is cyclical; that is, the components of the nursing process follow a logical sequence, but more than one component may be involved at any one time. The five components of the nursing process are the following:

1. *Assessing*—collecting, organizing, validating, and documenting data about a client's health status to establish a database. Activities include obtaining a health history, performing a physical assessment, reviewing client records, reviewing literature, and consulting support people and health professionals.
2. *Diagnosing*—the process of analyzing and synthesizing data, which results in a diagnostic statement or nursing diagnosis. Activities include clustering data; comparing data against standards; generating tentative hypotheses; identifying gaps and inconsistencies; determining the client's health strengths, risks, and problems; and formulating nursing diagnosis statements.
3. *Planning*—a series of steps in which the nurse and the client set priorities, goals, or desired outcomes

and establish a written care plan designed to resolve or minimize the identified problems of the client and to coordinate the care provided by all health team members. Activities include setting priorities with the client, writing evaluation goals and outcome criteria with the client, selecting nursing interventions, consulting with other health care personnel, writing nursing interventions and nursing care plans, and communicating the care plan to relevant health care providers.

4. *Implementing*—putting the nursing care plan into action to help the client attain goals. Activities include reassessing the client, updating the database, reviewing and revising the care plan, performing or delegating planned nursing interventions, and documenting nursing activities.
5. *Evaluating*—measuring the degree to which goals/outcomes have been achieved and identifying factors that promote or impede goal achievement. Activities include collecting data about the client's response, comparing the client's response to expected outcomes, relating nursing actions to client outcomes, drawing conclusions about problem status, and continuing, modifying, or terminating the care plan.

Refer to Chapters 10–14 of *Fundamentals of Nursing* for a thorough discussion of the components of the nursing process.

B. Aspects of Delegation

In nursing, delegation refers to indirect care—the intended outcome is achieved through the nursing work of someone supervised by the nurse—and involves defining the task, determining who can perform the task, describing the expectation, seeking agreement, monitoring performance, and providing feedback to the delegate regarding performance. The National Council of State Boards of Nursing published five "rights" of delegation: The nurse delegates the *right task,* under the *right circumstances,* to the *right person,* with the *right direction and communication,* and the *right supervision and evaluation* (National Council of State Boards of Nursing, 1997). Once the decision has been made to delegate, the nurse must communicate clearly and verify that the person understands the following:

- The specific tasks to be done for each client
- When each task is to be done
- The expected outcomes for each task including parameters outside of which an unlicensed person must immediately report to the nurse (and any action that must urgently be taken)
- Who is available to serve as a resource if needed
- When and in what format (written or verbal) a report on the tasks is expected

See Table 1–1 for examples of tasks that may and may not be delegated to unlicensed assistive personnel.

Table 1–1 Examples of Tasks That May and May Not Be Delegated to Unlicensed Assistive Personnel

Tasks That *May* Be Delegated to Unlicensed Assistive Personnel	Tasks That *May Not* Be Delegated to Unlicensed Assistive Personnel
• Taking vital signs • Measuring and recording intake and output • Client transfers and ambulation • Postmortem care • Bathing • Feeding • Gastrostomy feedings in established systems • Safety measures • Weighing • Simple dressing changes • Suction of chronic tracheostomies • Basic life support (cardio-pulmonary resuscitation)	• Assessment • Interpretation of data • Making a nursing diagnosis • Creation of a nursing care plan • Evaluation of care effectiveness • Care of invasive lines • Administering parenteral medications • Insertion of nasogastric tubes • Client education • Performing triage • Giving telephone advice

Principles Used by the Nurse to Determine Delegation to Unlicensed Assistive Personnel

1. The nurse must assess the individual client prior to delegating tasks.
2. The client must be medically stable or in a chronic condition and not fragile.
3. The task must be considered routine for this client.
4. The task must not require a substantial amount of scientific knowledge or technical skill.
5. The task must be considered safe for this client.
6. The task must have a predictable outcome.
7. Follow the agency's procedures and policies about delegation.

8. Know the scope of practice and the customary knowledge, skills, and job description for each health care discipline represented on your team.
9. Be aware of individual variations in work abilities. Along with different categories of caregivers are individual variations. Each individual has different experiences and may not be capable of performing every task cited in the job description.
10. When unsure about an assistant's abilities to perform a task, observe while the person performs it, or demonstrate it to the person and get a return demonstration before allowing the person to perform it independently.
11. Clarify reporting expectations to ensure the task is accomplished.
12. Create an atmosphere that fosters communication, teaching, and learning. For example, encourage staff to ask questions, listen carefully to their concerns, and make use of every opportunity to teach.

References

National Council of State Boards of Nursing. (1997). The five rights of delegation. Retrieved from https://www.ncsbn.org/Five_Rights_of_Delegation_NEW.pdf

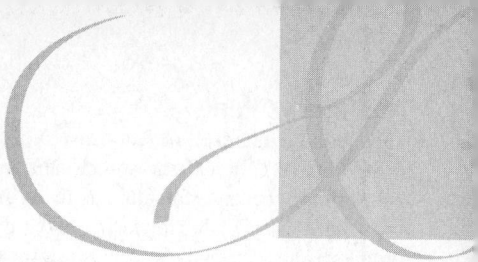

C. Communication Guidelines

Communication is a vital part of nursing practice. Nurses who communicate effectively are better able to initiate change that promotes health; establish a trusting relationship with clients, families, and colleagues; and prevent legal problems associated with nursing practice. Interpersonal attitudes are important. They convey beliefs, thoughts, and feelings about people and events. Attitudes such as caring, warmth, respect, and acceptance facilitate communication, whereas condescension, lack of interest, and coldness inhibit communication. Effective communication is essential to establishing a positive nurse–client relationship. Refer to Chapter 26 of *Fundamentals of Nursing* for a thorough discussion of communication techniques.

Therapeutic communication techniques can help promote understanding between nurse and client. These techniques include the following:

- Being silent when appropriate
- Asking open-ended questions
- Using touch when appropriate
- Restating or paraphrasing
- Seeking clarification
- Summarizing

In some situations, ordinary methods of communication are not sufficient: for example, when caring for a client who is angry, is confused, or speaks a language foreign to you. Some cultural issues also require sensitivity and understanding.

The Angry Client

Anger can be the result of fear, frustration, or a feeling of losing control. Often clients direct their anger toward the nurse, simply because the nurse is there. Angry outbursts from clients may be due to worries about their job, family, or illness. Fatigue or physical discomfort can also provoke anger. It is important that you try to identify the cause of the anger and not to feed that anger; maintain your composure.

The following are guidelines for responding to the angry client:

- Listen to what the client is saying.
- Do not let the client's anger cause you to react and not listen.
- Use techniques such as reflection, clarification, and focusing to determine the problem. Only when you understand the problem can you formulate a plan for resolution.
- Once the problem is identified, find ways to resolve it. Remember, **do not make promises you cannot keep.** A trusting relationship is key in diffusing angry outbursts.
- If you cannot resolve the client's anger, or if you feel any threat of violence, ask your instructor or the primary nurse for assistance.
- Be sure to document the conversation or incident, no matter how minor it may seem.

The Confused Client

Confusion in a client can be caused by medications, disease process, or the disruption of circadian rhythms. Whatever the cause, working with the confused client can be frustrating, so it is important to know your trigger points and what soothes them.

The following are guidelines for responding to the confused client:

- If this confusion is a new occurrence, review the client's medications and the potential side effects.

Sudden onset of confusion is a sign that *must* be reported. Review your findings with your instructor.

- At every interaction with the client, orient the client to person, time, and place. Try to interact with the client as often as possible.
- Actively listen to the client, and clarify any points of confusion. Be attentive.
- Ask the family to orient the client as well. Be sensitive to the family's needs; they too can become frustrated.
- Reassure the client, but do not be condescending.

The Anxious Client

Fear of the unknown causes anxiety. All of us experience it at one time or another. As a nurse, it is important that you identify the causes or origin of a client's fear or anxiety.

The following are guidelines to use in responding to the anxious client:

- Talk to the client and actively listen. Answer all questions you can answer accurately. Use the skills of reflection, clarification, and focusing to get the client to talk about the true problem.
- Questions such as "Am I going to die?" or "Do I have AIDS or cancer?" are the most disconcerting. Ask clients what makes them believe that they are going to die or that they have acquired immunodeficiency syndrome or cancer. Your goal is to get them to verbalize their fears.
- If the client has questions about the medical diagnosis, find out what the client has already been told. Clarify any points you can. If the client has not been told anything, ask whether the client would like to speak to the primary care provider. It is the primary care provider's responsibility, not yours, to communicate the diagnosis.
- Be attentive to the client. Check in on the client as much as possible. This establishes trust and communicates a caring attitude.

- Above all, do not be condescending or dismiss the client's anxiety. Put yourself in the client's position.

Communicating Across Language Barriers

There are many types of language barriers. Foreign language, hearing deficits, expressive disorders (e.g., aphasia), and intubation are all barriers to effective communication and require some creativity, patience, and perseverance. It is crucial for the client to be able to communicate needs and for the nurse to be able to communicate understanding. Health care facilities usually have resources that can help you, such as translation services for the non–English-speaking client and for the hearing-impaired. The speech therapy department can help you find ways to communicate with a client who has speech deficits.

The Non–English-Speaking Client

- Find out whether the health care facility has a translation service.
- Find out if any staff members speak the language.
- Do not yell at the client. Speaking more loudly may only make the client think you are angry. If the client does not understand English, increasing the decibel level does not help.
- If a particular language is commonly spoken at the facility (e.g., Spanish), purchase a phrase book and take the opportunity to add to your skills. You may also wish to develop a resource binder containing frequently used terms in many languages.
- If all else fails, act out what you are going to do. This does work.
- As a last resort, enlist the help of a family member or friend who may be able to translate. However, be considerate of these people; translating can be very stressful. Remember that they are the client's support system, not yours. Also, clients may be reluctant to share intimate health information with family members.

The Hearing-Impaired Client

- Stand in front of the hearing-impaired client and talk distinctly at a normal tone. Make sure the client can clearly see you. Many clients who are hard-of-hearing read lips.
- Keep paper and pencil at the bedside and write notes, especially when privacy is important.
- For the client who uses sign language, enlist the help of a translation service, if available.
- If no services are available to help you and writing is not possible, act out what you would like to do.
- Take the opportunity to learn sign language.

The Client with Aphasia

- Listen carefully. Encourage clients to take their time. Do not be afraid to ask clients to repeat themselves.
- Use paper and pencil, or picture board, if appropriate.
- If the aphasia is a long-standing condition, ask a family member for assistance.
- Call the speech therapy department for any additional help, if needed.

The Intubated Client

- Use paper and pencil for communication or a letter board on which the client can spell out words.
- If yes-or-no answers are needed, have the client blink once for yes and twice for no.

Cultural Issues

In almost every area of the country, nurses come into contact with people from cultures different from their own. Although it is not within the scope of this book to describe the differences in all cultures you may encounter, some universal guidelines can be of help.

Examine your own attitudes. What are your attitudes toward different cultures? What experiences have you had with different races and ethnic groups? What influences your acceptance or nonacceptance of a cultural group? Are your beliefs about a certain culture based on experience or on what you have heard or read? Refer to Chapter 18 of *Fundamentals of Nursing* for a thorough discussion of cultural issues.

The following are guidelines for responding to clients of different cultures:

- Always treat the client with respect.
- Different cultures may use different behaviors to denote respect or understanding. Do not assume you know the meaning of a specific behavior.
- Familiarize yourself with the customs and beliefs of cultural groups in your area.
- Try to incorporate cultural symbols and practices into the care plan of the client where feasible; these can bring comfort to a client.
- Remember that the color of a person's skin does not necessarily indicate the person's cultural background.
- Learn how the client views health, illness, grieving, and the health care system.

Special Care for Older Adults

Communication

It is important that health care providers who work with older adults increase their awareness of and avoid the use of *elderspeak.* Elderspeak is a speech style similar to baby talk. It does not communicate respect, but instead gives the message of dependence and incompetence to older adults. The characteristics of elderspeak include the following:

- Inappropriate terms of endearment (e.g., honey, sweetie)
- Inappropriate plural nouns (e.g., "Are *we* ready for *our* medicine?)

- Tag questions that prompt the answer and imply that the elder cannot act alone (e.g., "You would rather wear the blue shirt, *wouldn't you*?")
- Baby talk instead of the usual sentence structure, speech rate, and vocabulary

Older adults may have physical or cognitive problems that necessitate nursing interventions for improvement of communication skills. Some of the common ones are the following:

- Sensory deficits, such as vision and hearing
- Cognitive impairment, as in dementia
- Neurologic deficits from strokes or other neurologic conditions, such as aphasia (expressive and/or receptive) and lack of movement
- Psychosocial problems, such as depression

Recognizing specific needs and obtaining appropriate resources for clients can greatly increase their socialization and quality of life. Interventions directed toward improving communication in clients with these special needs are the following:

- Ensuring that assistive devices, glasses, and hearing aids are being used and are in good working order
- Making referrals to appropriate resources, such as speech therapy
- Making use of communications aids, such as communication boards, computers, and pictures, when possible
- Keeping environmental distractions to a minimum
- Speaking in short, simple sentences, one subject at a time—reinforce or repeat what is said when necessary
- Always facing the person when speaking—coming up behind someone may be frightening
- Including family and friends in conversation

- Using reminiscing, either in individual conversations or in groups to maintain memory connections and to enhance self-identity and self-esteem in the elder
- Believing the nonverbal when verbal expression and nonverbal expression are incongruent (Clarification of this and attentiveness to the elder's feelings help promote a feeling of caring and acceptance.)
- Finding out what has been important and has meaning to the person and trying to maintain these things as much as possible (Even simple things such as bedtime rituals become important if he or she is lost in a hospital or extended-care setting.)

Communication Among Health Professionals

Effective communication among the health professions is as important as the promotion of therapeutic communication between the nurse and the client. Skilled communication is critical for a number of situations: preserving a nurse's professional integrity while ensuring a client's safety, during nurse and physician communication, and at change-of-shift reporting.

Communication problems among health care professionals can cause disruptive behavior. The Center for American Nurses (2008) defines disruptive behavior as "behavior that interferes with effective communication among health-care providers and negatively impacts performance and outcomes." Disruptive behavior is not supportive of a culture of safety. Three common disruptive behaviors reported among nurses are incivility, lateral violence, and bullying.

As a result, nurses need to be as proficient in communication skills as they are in clinical skills. The American Association of Critical-Care Nurses developed standards for establishing and sustaining health work environments. The association's communication standard includes the following critical elements for the nurse (American Association of Critical-Care Nurses, 2005):

- Skilled communicators focus on finding solutions and achieving desirable outcomes.
- Skilled communicators seek to protect and advance collaborative relationships among colleagues.
- Skilled communicators invite and hear all relevant perspectives.
- Skilled communicators call upon goodwill and mutual respect to build consensus and arrive at common understanding.
- Skilled communicators demonstrate congruence between words and actions, holding others accountable for doing the same.
- Skilled communicators have access to appropriate communications technologies and are proficient in their use.

The above critical elements for skilled communication preserve a nurse's professional integrity while ensuring a client's safety.

1. SBAR Communication Guidelines

Few guidelines exist for the frequent verbal communication that occurs between nurses and doctors. One model, called SBAR (situation, background, assessment, recommendations), provides a standardized framework for communicating important information.

The SBAR format can be used by nurses in almost all forms of communication, including when calling a physician or other health care provider about a change in a client's condition, for shift reports, giving reports on clients being transferred within or outside the health facility, and sending clients for procedures. Box 1–1 contains more details on this communication framework.

Box 1–1 SBAR: Situation, Background, Assessment, Recommendation Model

A FRAMEWORK FOR NURSE–PHYSICIAN COMMUNICATION

S = Situation: What is the situation you are calling about? Provide your name, health agency, client name, and brief information about the problem.

B = Background: Information pertinent to the current situation, such as admitting diagnosis, date of admission, and important clinical information that relates to the call.

A = Assessment: This refers to what the nurse thinks is going on. If unsure of the problem, try to determine which body system is involved. Indicate the severity of the problem.

R = Recommendation: What is your recommendation for resolving the problem or what do you need from the health care provider (e.g., come see the client, transfer to another unit, or an order for a medication).

EXAMPLE OF USING SBAR WHEN CALLING A HEALTH CARE PROVIDER ABOUT A CLIENT PROBLEM

S: Health care provider called. Nurse has given name and unit of health care agency. "I'm calling about Sally Somers, a 19-year-old admitted this morning with a ruptured appendix. She is now 6 hours postop and has not voided.

B: Her bladder is distended. She is complaining of urgency to void but unable to do so even with sitting on commode, running water, etc. Everything else is stable.

A: She is very uncomfortable and crying because of her urinary retention.

R: "Could you give an order for a straight urinary catheterization?"

From "Raising the SBAR. How Better Communication Improves Patient Outcomes." B. B. Pope, L. Rodzen, and G. Spross, 2008, *Nursing*, 38(3), pp. 41–43.

Prepare before calling the primary care provider to report a client problem. You will be using the SBAR method. However, you also need to think about what information may be asked of you and be prepared to answer those questions. This means knowing the most recent client assessment data, including vital signs, lab data, and other tests, if appropriate. Have the client's medical record, MAR, and other flow sheets as needed available to you.

2. Handoff Communication/ Change-of-Shift Report

A hospital is required to implement a standardized approach to "handoff" communication, which is a process where information about patient/client/resident care is communicated in a consistent manner. Hospital handoffs occur at many times, including but not limited to change-of-shift reports, client transfer between units, and discharge. Box 1–2 lists the elements of performance required for effective handoff communication.

The change-of-shift report is given to all nurses on the next shift. Its purposes are to provide continuity of care for clients by providing critical information and to promote client safety and best practices. The nurse must focus on the needs of the client and not become distracted by irrelevant information. See Box 1–3.

Box 1–2 Key Elements for Effective Handoff Communication

The communication should include the following:

- Up-to-date information
- Interactive communication allowing for questions between the giver and receiver of client information
- Method for verifying the information (e.g., repeat-back, read-back techniques)
- Minimal interruptions
- Opportunity for receiver of information to review relevant client data (e.g., previous care and treatment)

Box 1–3 Focusing on Relevant Information During a Change-of-Shift Report

- Follow a particular order (e.g., follow room numbers in a hospital).
- Provide basic identifying information for each client (e.g., name, room number, bed designation). Report information in the same order every time.
- For new clients, provide the reason for admission or medical diagnosis (or diagnoses), surgery (date), diagnostic tests, and therapies in past 24 hours.
- Include significant changes in client's condition and present information in order (i.e., assessment, nursing diagnoses, interventions, outcomes, and evaluation). For example, "Mr. Ronald Oakes said he had an aching pain in his left calf at 1400 hours. Inspection revealed no other signs. Calf pain is related to altered blood circulation. Rest and elevation of his legs on a footstool for 30 minutes provided relief."
- Provide exact information, such as "Ms. Jessie Jones received morphine 6 mg IV at 1500 hours," not "Ms. Jessie Jones received some morphine during the evening."
- Report clients' need for special emotional support. For example, a client who has just learned that his biopsy results revealed malignancy and who is now scheduled for a laryngectomy needs time to discuss his feelings before preoperative teaching is begun.
- Include current nurse-prescribed and primary care provider-prescribed orders.
- Clearly state priorities of care and care that is due after the shift begins. For example, in a 7 AM report the nurse might say, "Mr. Li's vital signs are due at 0730, and his IV bag will need to be replaced by 0800." Give this information at the end of that client's report, because memory is best for the first and last information given.
- Be concise. Don't elaborate on background data and routine care (e.g., do not report "Vital signs at 0800 and 1150" when that is the unit standard). Do not report coming and going of visitors unless there is a problem or concern, or visitors are involved in teaching and care. Social support and visits are the norm.

- Incorporate a verification process (e.g., opportunity to ask and respond) to ensure that information is both received and understood.

3. Telephone and Verbal Orders

Primary care providers often order a therapy (e.g., medication order) for a client by telephone. Most agencies have specific policies about telephone orders. Many agencies allow only registered nurses to take telephone orders. While the primary care provider gives the telephone order:

- Write the complete order down on the physician's order form.
- Read it back to the primary care provider to ensure accuracy.
- Question any order that is ambiguous, unusual, or contraindicated by the client's condition.
- Have the primary care provider verbally acknowledge the read-back of the verbal/telephone order.
- Indicate on the physician's order form that it is a verbal order (VO) or telephone order (TO). See Box 1–4 for selected guidelines.

Box 1–4 Guidelines for Telephone and Verbal Orders

1. Know the state nursing board's position on who can give and accept verbal and phone orders.
2. Know the agency's policy regarding phone orders (e.g., colleague listens on extension and cosigns order sheet).
3. Ask the prescriber to speak slowly and clearly.
4. Ask the prescriber to spell out the medication if you are not familiar with it.
5. Question the drug, dosage, or changes if they seem inappropriate for this client.
6. Write the order down or enter into a computer on the physician's order form.

(*continued*)

Box 1–4 Guidelines for Telephone and Verbal Orders (*continued*)

7. Read the order back to the prescriber. Use words instead of abbreviations (e.g., three times a day for tid).
8. Have the prescriber verbally acknowledge the readback (e.g., "Yes, that is correct").
9. Record date and time and indicate it was a telephone order (TO). Sign name and credentials.
10. When writing a dosage always put a number before a decimal (e.g., 0.3 mL) but never after a decimal (e.g., 6 mg).
11. Write out units (e.g., 15 units of insulin, not 15 u of insulin).
12. Transcribe the order.
13. Follow agency protocol about the prescriber's protocol for signing telephone orders (e.g., within 24 hours).

Other:

- Never follow a voice-mail order. Call the prescriber for a client order. Write it down and read it back for confirmation.

References

American Association of Critical-Care Nurses. (2005). *AACN standards for establishing and sustaining healthy work environments: A journey to excellence*. Aliso Viejo, CA: Author.

Center for American Nurses. (2008). Lateral violence and bullying in the workplace. Retrieved from http://www.centerforamericannurses.org/associations/9102/files/Position%20StatementLateral%20Violence%20and%20Bullying.pdf

Pope, B. B., Rodzen, L., & Spross, G. (2008). Raising the SBAR. How better communication improves patient outcomes. *Nursing, 38*(3), 41–43.

UNIT 2

ASSESSMENT AND DIAGNOSIS

A. Nursing Health History
B. Methods of Examining
C. Vital Signs
D. Physical Health Examination
E. Nursing Diagnoses

A. Nursing Health History

The nursing health history is the first part of the assessment of the client's health status. Through this structured interview, you collect specific health data and obtain a detailed health record of the client. The client is the primary source of information.

You may also consult other sources for information about the client's health, including the medical record if available, and consultations with members of the health care team, family members, or significant others. It is important to be systematic in your approach and document your findings.

Before starting the interview, be sure to introduce yourself and state your purpose for collecting data. Establish rapport to put the client at ease and facilitate the interview process.

Biographic Data

- Obtain client's name, address, age, sex, marital status, occupation, religious preference, and usual source of medical care.

Chief Complaint or Reason for Visit

- The answer given to the question "What is troubling you?" or "Describe the reason you came to the hospital or clinic today." is the chief complaint, which should be recorded in the client's own words.

History of Present Illness

- When the symptoms started
- Whether the onset of symptoms was sudden or gradual

- How often the problem occurs
- Exact location of the distress
- Character of the complaint (e.g., intensity of pain or quality of sputum, emesis, or discharge)
- Activity in which the client was involved when the problem occurred
- Phenomena or symptoms associated with the chief complaint
- Factors that aggravate or alleviate the problem

Past History

- Childhood illnesses, such as chickenpox, mumps, measles, rubella (German measles), rubeola (red measles), streptococcal infections, scarlet fever, rheumatic fever, and other significant illnesses
- Immunizations and date of the last tetanus shot
- Allergies to foods, drugs, animals, insects, or other environmental agents, the type of reaction that occurs, and how the reaction is treated
- Injuries: how, when, and where the incident occurred; type of injury; treatment received; and any complications
- Hospitalization for serious illnesses: reasons for the hospitalization, dates, surgery performed, course of recovery, and any complications
- Medications: all currently used prescription and over-the-counter medications, such as aspirin, nasal spray, vitamins, or laxatives; herbs; and homeopathic remedies

Family History of Illness

- Ages of siblings, parents, and grandparents and their current state of health or the cause of death (if they are deceased); particular attention to disorders such as heart disease, cancer, diabetes, hypertension, obesity, allergies, arthritis, tuberculosis, bleeding, alcoholism, and any mental health disorders

Lifestyle

- Personal habits: the amount, frequency, and duration of substance use (tobacco, alcohol, coffee, cola, tea, and illicit or recreational drugs)
- Diet: description of a typical diet on a normal day or any special diet, number of meals and snacks per day, who cooks and shops for food, ethnic food patterns, and allergies
- Sleep/rest patterns: usual daily sleep/wake times, difficulties sleeping, and remedies used for difficulties
- Activities of daily living: any difficulties experienced in the basic activities of eating, grooming, dressing, elimination, and locomotion
- Instrumental activities of daily living: any difficulties experienced in food preparation, shopping, transportation, housekeeping, laundry, and ability to use the telephone, handle finances, and manage medications
- Recreation/hobbies: exercise activity and tolerance, hobbies and other interests, and vacations

Social Data

- Family relationships/friendships: the client's support system (those who help in time of need), effect the client's illness has on the family, whether any family problems are affecting the client
- Ethnic affiliation: health customs and beliefs; cultural practices that may affect health care and recovery
- Educational history: data about the client's highest level of education attained and any past difficulties with learning
- Occupational history: current employment status, days missed from work because of illness, history of accidents on the job, occupational hazards with a potential for future disease or accident, client's need to change jobs because of past illness, employment status of spouses or partners and the way child care is handled, and client's overall satisfaction with work

- Economic status: how the client pays for medical care (including what kind of medical and hospitalization coverage the client has) and whether the client's illness presents financial concerns
- Home and neighborhood conditions: home safety measures and adjustments in physical facilities that may be required to help the client manage physical disability, activity intolerance, and activities of daily living; availability of neighborhood and community services to meet the client's needs

Psychological Data

- Major stressors experienced and the client's perception of them
- Usual coping pattern with a serious problem or a high level of stress
- Communication style: ability to verbalize appropriate emotion; nonverbal communication such as eye movements, gestures, use of touch, and posture; interactions with support persons; and congruence of nonverbal behavior and verbal expression

Patterns of Health Care

- Health care resources the client is currently using and has used in the past. These include primary care provider, specialists (e.g., ophthalmologist or gynecologist), dentist, folk practitioners (e.g., herbalist or curandero), health clinic, or health center; whether the client considers the care being provided adequate; and whether access to health care is a problem

Review of Systems

The goal of the review of systems is to gather subjective data from the client on each of the major body systems.

- *General health.* Weight loss, weakness, feelings of fatigue, mood changes, night sweats, or bleeding tendencies?
- *Skin.* Skin diseases such as eczema, psoriasis, acne; change in pigmentation; tendency toward bruising;

excessive dryness or moisture; jaundice; itching, rashes, hives; change in color or size of moles; or open sores that are slow to heal?

- *Hair.* Itchy scalp, loss of hair, excessive body hair? Does the client wear a wig?
- *Nails.* Color changes, biting, clubbing, splitting?
- *Head.* Frequent or severe headaches, fainting, dizziness, accident resulting in unconsciousness?
- *Eyes.* Difficulty seeing, eye infection, eye pain, excessive tearing, double vision, blurring, sensitivity to light, cataracts, itching, spots in front of eyes? Does the client wear glasses (for near or far vision) or contact lenses? When was the client's last eye examination?
- *Ears.* Any infection, loss of hearing, pain, discharge, ringing in the ears? Does the client wear a hearing aid?
- *Nose.* Frequent colds, nosebleeds, allergies, pain, tenderness, postnasal drip?
- *Mouth and throat.* Sore gums; bleeding gums; sores, lumps or white spots on mouth, lips, or tongue; toothaches, cavities, or difficulty swallowing; voice change or hoarseness? Does the client wear dentures (upper, lower, partial)? When was the client's last dental appointment?
- *Neck.* Pain, swelling, stiffness, limited movement, swollen glands?
- *Breasts.* Nipple discharge, scaling or cracks around nipples, dimples, lumps, pattern of breast self-examination? Last mammogram?
- *Respiratory system.* Chest pain; cough; shortness of breath; wheezing; coughing up blood; lung disease such as tuberculosis, emphysema, asthma, or bronchitis? Has the client ever had a chest x-ray? When? Results?
- *Cardiovascular system.* Heart disease, palpitations, heart murmur, high blood pressure, anemia, varicose veins, leg swelling or ulcer?
- *Gastrointestinal system.* Nausea, vomiting, loss of appetite, indigestion, heartburn, bright blood in stools,

tarry-black stools, diarrhea, constipation, abdominal pain, excessive gas, hemorrhoids, rectal pain, colostomy, ileostomy?

- *Genitourinary system.* Frequency, dribbling, urgency, urination at night, difficulty starting stream, blood in urine, incontinence, pain or burning upon urination, urinary tract infection, ureterostomy, sexually transmitted infection such as gonorrhea or syphilis?
  - *Females:* Age of menarche, last menstrual period, duration, amount of flow, regularity of cycle? Any problems with painful menstruation, bleeding between periods, pain during intercourse, vaginal discharge, vaginal itching, vaginal infection?
  - *Males:* Penile discharge, swelling, masses or lesions, difficulty in sexual functioning?
- *Musculoskeletal system.* Muscular pain, swelling, or weakness; joint swelling, soreness, or stiffness; leg cramps; bone defects?
- *Neurologic system.* Difficulty walking; unconsciousness; seizures; tremors; paralysis; numbness, tingling, or burning sensations in any body part; weakness on one side of body; speech problems; loss of memory; disorientation; forgetfulness; unclear thinking; changes in emotional state?
- *Endocrine system.* History of goiter, heat or cold intolerance, diabetes, excessive thirst, excessive eating?

B. Methods of Examining

The four primary techniques used in the physical examination are inspection, palpation, percussion, and auscultation.

Inspection

Inspection, or visual examination, should be done systematically, with sufficient light.

Palpation

Palpation is the use of the sense of touch to determine texture, temperature, vibration, position, size, consistency, mobility, distention, pulsation, and tenderness or pain.

Percussion

In percussion, the body surface is struck to elicit sounds that can be heard or vibrations that can be felt.

Percussion is used to determine the size and shape of the internal organs by establishing their borders. It indicates whether tissue is fluid-filled, air-filled, or solid. Percussion elicits five types of sounds:

- Flatness (extremely dull)—bone and muscle
- Dullness (thudlike)—liver, spleen, heart
- Resonance (hollow)—air-filled lung
- Hyperresonance (booming)—emphysematous lung
- Tympany (drumlike)—air-filled stomach

The two types of percussion methods are direct/immediate and indirect/mediate.

Direct Percussion

- Strike the area to be percussed with two or more fingers, using the pads of the fingers only.
- Use rapid wrist movements.

Indirect Percussion

- Place the middle finger of your nondominant hand firmly on the skin of the area to be percussed. (Use only the distal phalanx and joint of the finger.)
- Using the flexed middle finger of the dominant hand, strike the middle finger of the nondominant hand. Be sure to use rapid wrist movements.

Auscultation

Auscultation is the process of listening to sounds produced within the body. The use of an unaided ear is the direct method of auscultation. The use of a stethoscope is considered an indirect method. Auscultated sounds are described according to the following:

- Pitch—frequency of vibrations
- Intensity—loudness or softness
- Duration—length of the sound
- Quality—subjective description of the sound

C. Vital Signs

Vital signs are obtained to monitor the functions of the body. The temperature, pulse, respiratory rate, blood pressure, and oxygen concentration measurements indicate how the body is functioning or responding to medications or treatments. Refer to Chapter 29 of *Fundamentals of Nursing* for a thorough discussion of vital signs. Pain is also one of the vital signs. See Unit 3, Clinical Guidelines 2, for details on pain assessment and treatment.

Temperature

Temperature is a measurement of the balance between heat produced by the body and heat lost from the body. A fever results from inadequate heat loss; a low temperature results from excessive heat loss. When measured orally, adult temperature is 36°C to 37.5°C. Leave the thermometer in place for the length of time recommended for the type of thermometer and location of measurement. Temperatures can be taken via the following methods:

- Oral—If the client is too young, confused, or unable to cooperate, use another means of measuring temperature.
- Rectal—Use water-soluble lubricant to insert the thermometer. Do not use the rectal method if client has rectal disease or convulsions. Be sure to hold a child firmly.
- Axillary—Wipe the axillary area if damp. After placing the thermometer, hold the arm against the chest.
- Tympanic membrane—Readily accessible; very fast.
- Temporal artery—Safe and noninvasive; very fast.

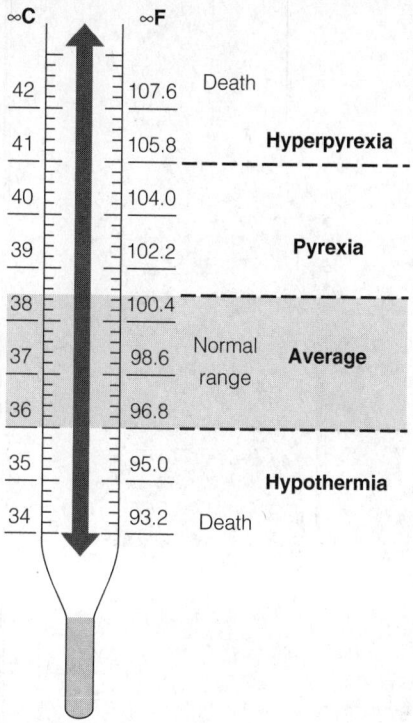

Pulse

The pulse is a wave of blood created by contraction of the heart's left ventricle. See Figure 2–1 for pulse sites.

To take a client's pulse, proceed with the following steps:

- Before taking the pulse, ensure that the client is at rest. If the client has been active, wait 10 to 15 minutes.
- Use your index and middle fingers to palpate all pulse sites, except for the apex of the heart, where a stethoscope is required.
- Note rate, rhythm, volume, arterial wall elasticity, presence of bilateral equality, and intensity.
- Count irregular pulses a full 60 seconds.

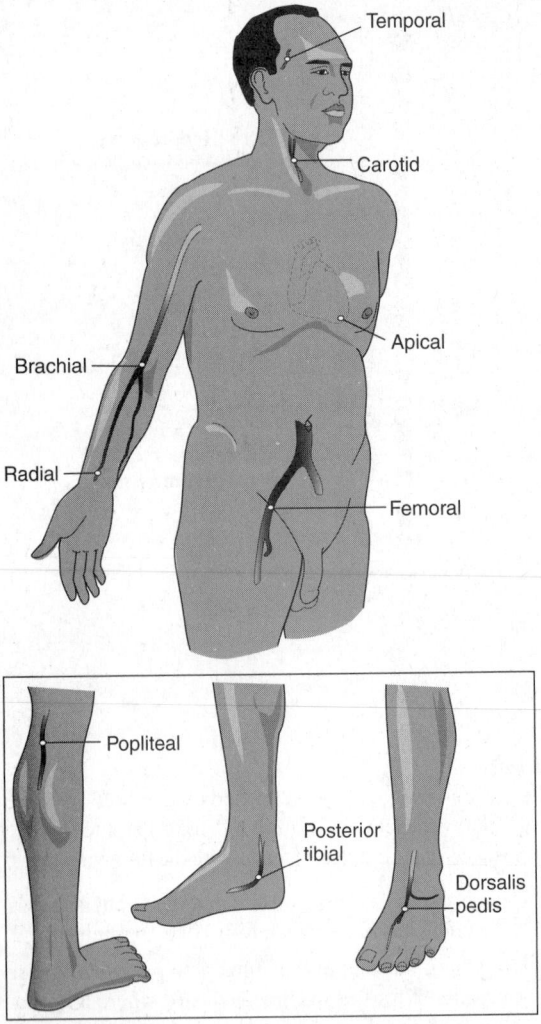

Figure 2–1 ■ Nine sites for taking pulses.

Respirations

When assessing respirations, note the rate (breaths per minute), depth (normal, deep, or shallow), rhythm (regularity), and quality (effort required to breathe, and the sound of the respirations). When possible, use the following methods to assess respirations, when the client is unaware that you are doing so:

- While standing at the bedside, ask the client to place the arm across the chest. The arm will rise and fall as the client breathes, making it easier to count respirations.
- After assessing the pulse, continue holding the wrist. Raise your eyes slightly to observe the chest.

Variations in Pulse and Respirations by Age

Age	Pulse Average (and Ranges)	Respirations Average (and Ranges)
Newborn	130 (80–180)	35 (30–60)
1 year	120 (80–140)	30 (20–40)
5–8 years	100 (75–120)	20 (15–25)
10 years	70 (50–90)	19 (15–25)
Teen	75 (50–90)	18 (15–20)
Adult	80 (60–100)	16 (12–20)
Older adult	70 (60–100)	16 (15–20)

Blood Pressure

Blood pressure is a measure of the pressure the blood exerts as it flows through the arteries. The systolic pressure (the top number) measures the amount of pressure during contraction of the ventricles, and the diastolic pressure (the bottom number) is the measure of the pressure in the arteries when the ventricles are at rest. Blood pressures can be taken on the arm or on the thigh. Points to remember include the following:

- Be sure the cuff is of adequate size. For the obese client, use a large or thigh cuff. The cuff should be wide enough to cover two-thirds of the limb.
- Make sure the client is calm and has not smoked or exercised within 30 minutes of the measurement.

- Inspect the arm or thigh before placing the cuff. Do not use an extremity that has an IV line or is injured.
- Position the limb so the artery is at heart level.
- If the client is sitting, both feet should be placed flat on the floor.
- Use the bell side of the amplifier of the stethoscope over the pulse site.
- Pump up the cuff until the sphygmomanometer reads 30 mm Hg above the point where the pulse disappeared.
- Release the valve on the cuff so that the pressure decreases at the rate of 2 to 3 mm Hg per second. Note the readings at Korotkoff phase 1 (first faint, clear tapping or thumping sounds), phase 4 (muffled and soft, blowing quality), and phase 5 (last sound is heard). Record as phase 1/phase 5 or phase 1/phase 4/phase 5, depending on agency policy.
- Wait 1 to 2 minutes before making further determinations.
- If this is the client's initial examination, repeat the procedure on the client's other limb.

Oxygen Saturation

A pulse oximeter is a noninvasive device that estimates a client's arterial blood oxygen saturation (SaO_2) by means of a sensor attached to the client's finger, toe, nose, earlobe, or forehead and reports a percent SpO_2.

- Choose a sensor appropriate for the client's weight, size, and desired location.
- If the client is allergic to adhesive, use a clip or sensor without adhesive. If using an extremity, assess the proximal pulse and capillary refill at the point closest to the site.
- Clean the site with an alcohol wipe before applying the sensor. It may be necessary to remove dark nail polish because it can interfere with accurate measurements or position the sensor on the side of the finger rather than perpendicular to the nail bed.

- Attach the sensor cable to the connection outlet on the oximeter (unless a wireless device is used).
- When using continuous monitoring, check the alarm limits for high and low oxygen saturation and high and low pulse rates. Oxygen saturation should be between 95%–100%.
- Inspect the location of an adhesive sensor every 4 hours and a spring-tension sensor every 2 hours.
- If indicated, cover the sensor with a sheet or towel to block large amounts of light from external sources (e.g., sunlight, procedure lamps, or bilirubin lights in the nursery).

D. Physical Health Examination

A complete health assessment is generally conducted starting from the head and moving toward the toes; however, the procedure can vary in many ways according to the age of the individual, the severity of the illness, the preferences of the nurse, and the agency's priorities and procedures. Regardless of what procedure is used, the client's energy and time must be considered. The health assessment is therefore conducted in a systematic and efficient manner that requires the fewest position changes for the client.

Frequently, nurses assess a specific body area instead of the entire body. These specific assessments are made in relation to client complaints, the nurse's own observation of the problem, the client's presenting problem, nursing interventions provided, and medical therapies.

While you are assessing the client, do not be afraid to talk and ask questions. Conversation puts the client at ease and gives you valuable subjective information.

Preparing the Client

Most people need an explanation of the physical health examination. Explain when and where the examination will take place, why it is necessary, who will conduct it, and what will happen during the examination. Also inform the client of any special circumstances—for instance, the need to go to a different room or assume a special position—and tell the client that appropriate draping will be provided so that the body will not be unnecessarily exposed.

Most clients should empty the bladder before the examination. Doing so helps them feel more relaxed and facilitates palpation of the abdomen and pubic area. If a urinalysis is required, urine should be collected in a container for that purpose.

Before you start, be sure to do the following:

- Collect your equipment.
- Explain to the client what you will be doing and approximately how long it will take to complete the examination. Establishing rapport with the client makes for a more relaxed examination for both of you.
- Cleanse your hands. Follow infection control precautions throughout.
- Ensure that the client's privacy is protected. Draw the curtain if the room is semiprivate.

Assessing the Client

General Survey

Appearance

- Observe body build, height, and weight in relation to the client's age, lifestyle, and health.
- Observe the client's posture and gait, standing, sitting, and walking.
- Observe the client's overall hygiene and grooming. Relate these to the person's activities before the assessment.
- Note body and breath odor in relation to activity level.
- Observe for signs of distress in posture (e.g., bending over because of abdominal pain) or facial expressions (e.g., wincing or labored breathing).
- Note obvious signs of health or illness (e.g., in skin color or breathing).

Mental Status

- Assess the client's attitude.
- Note the client's affect/mood; assess the appropriateness of the client's responses.

- Listen for quantity of speech (amount and pace), quality (loudness, clarity, inflection), and organization (coherence of thought, overgeneralization, vagueness).
- Listen for relevance and organization of thoughts.

The Integument

Skin

- Inspect skin color (best assessed under natural lighting and on areas not exposed to the sun).
- Inspect uniformity of skin color.
- Assess edema if present (e.g., location, color, temperature, shape, and the number of millimeters to which the skin remains indented or pitted when pressed by a finger).
- Inspect, palpate, and describe skin lesions. Palpate lesions to determine shape and texture. Describe lesions according to location, distribution, color, configuration, size, shape, type, or structure.
- Observe and palpate skin moisture.
- Palpate skin temperature. Compare the two feet and two hands using the backs of your fingers.
- Note skin turgor (fullness or elasticity) by lifting and pinching the skin on an extremity or over the sternum.

Hair

- Inspect the distribution of growth over the scalp.
- Inspect hair thickness or thinness, texture, and oiliness.
- Note the presence of infections or infestations by parting the hair in several areas.
- Inspect amount of body hair.

Nails

- Inspect nail plate shape to determine its curvature and angle.
- Inspect nail texture.
- Inspect nail color.
- Inspect tissues surrounding nails.

The Head

The Skull and Face

- Inspect the skull for size, shape, and symmetry.
- Palpate the skull for masses, depressions, or nodules.
- Inspect the facial features (e.g., symmetry of structures).
- Inspect the eyes for edema and hollowness.
- Note symmetry of facial movements. Ask the client to elevate the eyebrows, frown or lower the eyebrows, close the eyes tightly, puff the cheeks, and smile and show teeth.

The Eyes and Vision

External Eye Structures

- Inspect the eyebrows for hair distribution, alignment, skin quality, and movement (ask the client to raise and lower the eyebrows).
- Inspect the eyelashes for evenness of distribution and direction of the curl.
- Inspect the eyelids for surface characteristics such as skin quality and texture, position in relation to the cornea, ability to blink, and frequency of blinking.
- Inspect the bulbar conjunctiva (the conjunctiva lying over the sclera) for color, texture, and presence of lesions. Retract the eyelids and ask client to look up, down, and from side to side.
- Inspect the corneas for clarity and texture by using a penlight at an oblique angle to the eye.
- Inspect pupils for color, shape, and symmetry of size.
- Assess each pupil's direct and consensual reaction to light to determine the function of the third (oculomotor) and fourth (trochlear) cranial nerves.
- Assess each pupil's reaction to accommodation.

Visual Fields

- Assess peripheral visual fields to determine function of the retina and neuronal visual pathways to the brain and second (optic) cranial nerve.

Extraocular Muscle Tests

- Assess six ocular movements to determine eye alignment and coordination.
- Perform the cover-uncover patch test to determine eye alignment.
- Perform the corneal light reflex test to determine eye alignment.

Visual Acuity

- Assess near vision by asking the client to wear corrective lenses if used for reading. Ask the client to read from a document held 36 cm (14 in.) from the face.
- Assess distance vision using the Snellen or similar chart (with the client wearing corrective lenses if required, unless they are used for reading only).
- Perform functional vision tests (e.g., light perception, hand movements, counting fingers at 30 cm [1 foot]) if the client is unable to see the top line of the Snellen chart.

The Ears and Hearing

Auricles

- Inspect the auricles for color, symmetry of size, and position.
- Palpate the auricles for texture, elasticity, and areas of tenderness.

External Ear Canal and Tympanic Membrane

- Inspect the external ear canal for cerumen, skin lesions, pus, and blood. Using an otoscope, inspect the tympanic membrane for color.

Gross Hearing Acuity Test

- Assess client's response to normal voice tones.
- If the client has difficulty hearing the normal voice, perform the tuning fork tests.

Tuning Fork Tests

- Perform Weber's test to assess bone conduction.
- Perform the Rinne test to compare air conduction to bone conduction.

Nose and Sinuses

- Inspect the external nose for any deviations in shape, size, symmetry, or color. Inspect for flaring or discharge from the nares.
- Lightly palpate the external nose to determine any areas of tenderness, masses, and displacements of bone and cartilage.
- Inspect the nasal cavities using a penlight or a nasal speculum.
- Determine patency of both nasal cavities.
- Inspect the nasal cavities using a flashlight or a nasal speculum.
- Palpate the maxillary and frontal sinuses for tenderness.

The Mouth and Oropharynx

Lips and Buccal Mucosa

- Inspect the outer lips for symmetry of contour, color, and texture.
- Inspect and palpate the inner lips and buccal mucosa for color, moisture, texture, and the presence of lesions.

Teeth and Gums

- Inspect the teeth and gums while examining the inner lips and buccal mucosa.
- Inspect the dentures. Ask the client to remove complete or partial dentures. Inspect their condition, noting in particular broken or worn areas.

Tongue/Floor of Mouth

- Inspect the surface of the tongue for position, color, and texture by asking the client to protrude the tongue.
- Inspect tongue movement.
- Inspect the base of the tongue, the mouth floor, and the frenulum.

Palates and Uvula

- Inspect the hard palate and soft palate for color, shape, texture, and the presence of bony prominences.
- Inspect the uvula for position and mobility while examining the palates.

Oropharynx and Tonsils

- Inspect the oropharynx for color and texture.
- Inspect the tonsils for color, discharge, and size.

The Neck

Neck Muscles

- Inspect the neck muscles for abnormal swelling or masses.
- Observe head movement. Ask the client to move the chin to the chest, to move the head back so that the chin points upward, to move the head so that the ear is moved toward the shoulder on each side, and to turn the head to the right and to the left.
- Assess muscle strength by asking the client to turn the head against the resistance of your hand. Repeat with the other side. Then ask the client to shrug the shoulders against the resistance of your hands.

Lymph Nodes

- Palpate the entire neck for presence of enlarged lymph nodes.

Trachea

- Palpate the trachea for lateral deviation.

Thyroid Gland

- Inspect the thyroid gland by standing in front of the client.
- Observe the lower half of the neck overlying the thyroid gland for symmetry and visible masses.
- Ask the client to hyperextend the head and swallow to determine thyroid and cricoid movement.

The Thorax and Lungs

Posterior Thorax

- Inspect the shape and symmetry of the anterior, posterior, and lateral thorax.
- Inspect the spinal alignment for deformities.
- Palpate the posterior thorax.
- Palpate the posterior thorax for respiratory excursion.

- Palpate the thorax for vocal (tactile) fremitus, comparing each lung side.
- Percuss the thorax. Use a systematic zigzag procedure.
- Auscultate the thorax using the flat-disc diaphragm of the stethoscope. Ask the client to take slow, deep breaths through the mouth. Use a systematic zigzag procedure. Compare findings at each point with the corresponding point on the opposite side of the thorax. See Tables 2–1 and 2–2 for description of normal and adventitious breath sounds.

Anterior Thorax

- Inspect breathing patterns (e.g., respiratory rate and rhythm).
- Inspect the costal angle and the angle at which the ribs enter the spine.

Table 2–1 Normal Breath Sounds

Type	Description	Location	Characteristics
Vesicular	Soft-intensity, low-pitched, "gentle sighing" sounds created by air moving through smaller airways (bronchioles and alveoli)	Over peripheral lung; best heard at base of lungs	Best heard on inspiration, which is about 2.5 times longer than the expiratory phase (5:2 ratio)
Bronchovesicular	Moderate-intensity and moderate-pitched "blowing" sounds created by air moving through larger airway (bronchi)	Between the scapulae and lateral to the sternum at the first and second intercostal spaces	Equal inspiratory and expiratory phases (1:1 ratio)
Bronchial (tubular)	High-pitched, loud, "harsh" sounds created by air moving through the trachea	Anteriorly over the trachea; not normally heard over lung tissue	Louder than vesicular sounds; have a short inspiratory phase and long expiratory phase (1:2 ratio)

Table 2–2 Adventitious Breath Sounds

Name	Description	Cause	Location
Crackles (rales)	Fine, short, interrupted crackling sounds; alveolar rales are high-pitched. Sound can be simulated by rolling a lock of hair near the ear. Best heard on inspiration but can be heard on both inspiration and expiration. May not be cleared by coughing	Air passing through fluid or mucus in any air passage	Most commonly heard in the bases of the lower lung lobes
Gurgles (rhonchi)	Continuous, low-pitched, coarse, gurgling, harsh, louder sounds with a moaning or snoring quality. Best heard on expiration but can be heard on both inspiration and expiration. May be altered by coughing	Air passing through narrowed air passages as a result of secretions, swelling, tumors	Loud sounds can be heard over most lung areas but predominate over the trachea and bronchi
Friction rub	Superficial grating or creaking sounds heard during inspiration and expiration. Not relieved by coughing	Rubbing together of inflamed pleural surfaces	Heard most often in areas of greatest thoracic expansion (e.g., lower anterior and lateral chest)
Wheeze	Continuous, high-pitched, squeaky musical sounds. Best heard on expiration. Not usually altered by coughing	Air passing through a constricted bronchus as a result of secretions, swelling, tumors	Heard over all lung fields; best heard on expiration

- Palpate the anterior thorax for respiratory excursion and tactile fremitus.
- Percuss the anterior thorax symmetrically. Begin above the clavicles in the supraclavicular space, and proceed down to the diaphragm. Compare the lung on one side to the lung on the other side.
- Auscultate the trachea.
- Auscultate the anterior chest. Use the sequence used in percussion, beginning over the bronchi between the sternum and the clavicles. See Tables 2–1 and 2–2 for description of normal and adventitious breath sounds.

The Cardiovascular and Peripheral Vascular Systems

The Heart and Central Vessels

- Simultaneously inspect and palpate the precordium for the presence of abnormal pulsations, lifts, or heaves.
- Inspect and palpate the aortic, pulmonic, tricuspid, and mitral areas for pulsations.
- Inspect and palpate the apical area for pulsation, noting its specific location and diameter.
- Auscultate the heart in all four anatomic sites: aortic, pulmonic, tricuspid, and mitral. See Figure 2–2.
- Inspect and palpate the epigastric area (at the base of the sternum) for abdominal aortic pulsations.
- Palpate the carotid arteries one at a time.
- Auscultate the carotid artery to determine the presence of a bruit.
- Inspect the jugular veins for distention while the client is in a semi-Fowler's position with the head supported on a small pillow.

The Peripheral Vascular System

- Palpate the peripheral pulses on both sides of the client's body systematically and simultaneously to determine the symmetry of pulse volume. If you have difficulty palpating the peripheral pulses, use a Doppler ultrasound probe.

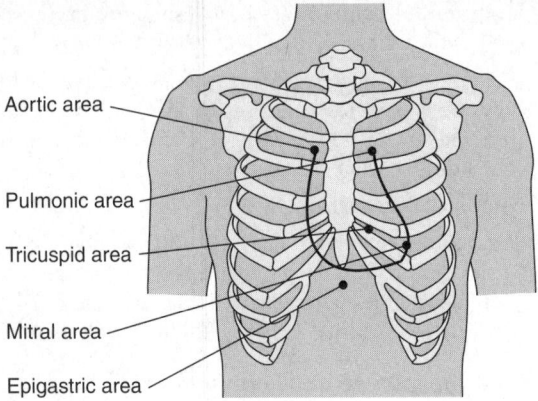

Figure 2–2 ■ Anatomic sites of the precordium.

Peripheral Veins

- Inspect the peripheral veins in the arms and legs for the presence or appearance of superficial veins when limbs are dependent and when limbs are elevated.
- Assess the peripheral leg veins for signs of phlebitis.

Peripheral Perfusion

- Inspect the skin of the hands and the feet for color, temperature, edema, and skin changes.
- Assess the adequacy of arterial flow if arterial insufficiency is suspected.

The Breasts and Axillae

- Use this as an opportunity to teach breast self-examination.
- Inspect and palpate the breasts of both men and women.
- Inspect the breasts for size, symmetry, and contour or shape while the client is in a sitting position.
- Inspect the skin of the breast for localized discolorations or hyperpigmentation, retraction or dimpling, localized hypervascular areas, swelling, or edema.

- Accentuate any retraction by having the client raise the arms above the head, push the hands together with elbows fixed, and/or press the hands down on the hips.
- Inspect the areola and nipple area for size, shape, symmetry, color, surface characteristics, and any masses or lesions.
- Palpate the axillary, subclavicular, and supraclavicular lymph nodes when the client is supine. Use the palmar surface of all fingertips to palpate.
- Palpate the breast for masses, tenderness, and any discharge from the nipples. Start at one point for palpation and move systematically to the end point to ensure that all breast surfaces are assessed.

The Abdomen

Inspection of the Abdomen

- Inspect the abdomen for skin integrity, contour, and symmetry.
- Observe abdominal movements associated with respiration, peristalsis, or aortic pulsations.
- Observe the vascular pattern.

Auscultation of the Abdomen

- Auscultate the abdomen for bowel sounds, vascular sounds, and peritoneal friction rubs in all four quadrants. See Figure 2–3.

Percussion of the Abdomen

- Percuss several areas in each of the four quadrants to determine presence of tympany (gas in stomach and intestines) and dullness (decrease, absence, or flatness of resonance over solid masses or fluid).

Palpation of the Abdomen

- Perform light palpation first to detect areas of tenderness and/or muscle guarding. Systematically explore all four quadrants.

Palpation of the Bladder

- Palpate the area above the pubic symphysis if the client's history indicates possible urinary retention.

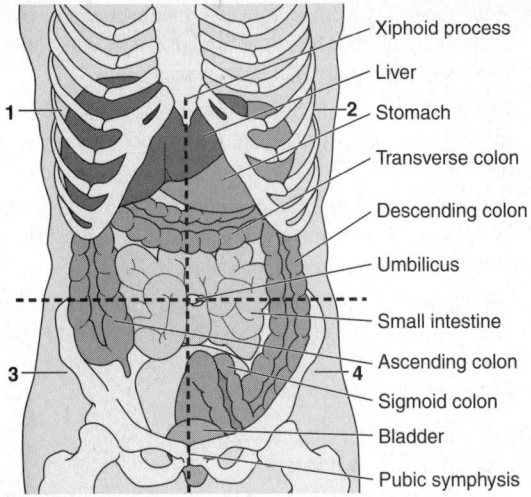

Figure 2–3 ■ The four abdominal quadrants and the underlying organs. *1,* right upper quadrant; *2,* left upper quadrant; *3,* right lower quadrant; *4,* left lower quadrant.

The Musculoskeletal System

The Muscles

- Inspect muscles for size. Compare the muscles on one side of the body to the corresponding muscles on the other side.
- Inspect muscles and tendons for contractures.
- Inspect the muscles for tremors. Inspect any tremors by having the client hold the arms out in front of the body.
- Test muscle strength. Compare the right side with the left side. Include shoulders, arms, hands, legs, and feet.

The Bones

- Inspect the skeleton for normal structure and deformities.
- Palpate the bones to locate any areas of edema or tenderness.

The Joints

- Inspect the joints for swelling.
- Palpate each joint for tenderness, smoothness of movement, swelling, crepitation, and the presence of nodules.
- Assess joint range of motion.

The Neurologic System

If not done previously, assess for language, orientation, memory, attention span and calculation, level of consciousness, cranial nerves, and reflexes.

Gross Motor and Balance Test

Of the several gross motor function and balance tests, generally Romberg's test and one other are conducted. The following tests may be carried out.

- Romberg test (Ask the client to stand with feet together and arms resting at the sides, first with eyes open, then closed. Stand close during this test to prevent the client from falling.)
- Standing on one foot with eyes closed
- Heel–toe walking
- Toe or heel walking

Fine Motor Tests for the Upper Extremities

The following tests may be performed:

- Finger to nose
- Alternating supination and pronation of hands on knees
- Finger to nose and to the nurse's finger
- Finger to fingers
- Fingers to thumb (same hand)

Fine Motor Tests for the Lower Extremities

Ask the client to lie supine and perform these tests:

- Heel down opposite shin. Ask the client to place the heel of one foot just below the opposite knee and run the heel down the shin to the foot. Repeat with the other foot.

- Toe or ball of foot to the nurse's finger. Ask the client to touch your finger with the large toe of each foot.

Sensory Function

- Light-touch sensation. Compare the light-touch sensation of symmetric areas of the body.
- Pain sensation. Assess pain sensation by asking the client to close the eyes and report whether a sharp, dull, or indistinguishable sensation is felt when you touch the skin with the sharp or dull end of an instrument. Alternate between the sharp and dull ends, and randomly select different anatomic sites. Do not perform this test on the face.

Position or Kinesthetic Sensation

- Commonly, the middle fingers and the large toes are tested for the kinesthetic sensation (sense of position).
- Ask the client to close the eyes. Move the finger or toe until it is up, down, or straight out, and ask the client to identify the position.

The Female Genitals and Inguinal Lymph Nodes

- Inspect the distribution, amount, and characteristics of pubic hair.
- Inspect the skin of the pubic area for lesions, swelling, inflammation, and presence of parasites. To assess adequately, separate the labia majora and labia minora.
- Inspect the clitoris, urethral orifice, and vaginal orifice when separating the labia minora.
- Palpate the inguinal lymph nodes using the pads of the fingers in a rotary motion, noting any enlargement or tenderness.

The Male Genitals and Inguinal Area

- Use this as an opportunity to teach testicular self-examination.
- Inspect pubic hair distribution, amount, and characteristics.
- Inspect the penile shaft and glans for lesions, nodules, swelling, and inflammation.

- Inspect the urethral meatus for swelling, inflammation, and discharge.
- Inspect the scrotum for appearance, size, and symmetry.
- Inspect inguinal areas for bulges while the client is standing, if possible. Have the client hold the breath and strain or bear down as though having a bowel movement.

The Rectum and Anus

- Inspect the anus and surrounding tissue for color, integrity, and skin lesions.

Special Considerations for Assessment of Older Adults

History

- Allow extra time for clients to answer questions.
- Adapt questioning techniques as appropriate for clients with hearing or visual limitations.
- Older adults can lose several inches in height. Be sure to document height and ask if they are aware of becoming shorter in height.
- When asking about weight loss, be specific about amount and time frame, e. g., "Have you lost more than five pounds in the last two months?"

The Skin

- Changes in white skin occur at an earlier age than in black skin.
- The skin loses its elasticity and wrinkles. Wrinkles first appear on the skin of the face and neck, which are abundant in collagen and elastic fibers.
- The skin appears thin and translucent because of loss of dermis and subcutaneous fat.
- The skin is dry and flaky because sebaceous and sweat glands are less active. Dry skin is more prominent over the extremities.
- The skin takes longer to return to its natural shape after being tented between the thumb and finger.

- Due to the normal loss of peripheral skin turgor in older adults, assess for hydration by checking skin turgor over the sternum or clavicle.
- *Senile lentigines* or *melanotic freckles* are normally apparent on the back of the hand and other skin areas that are exposed to the sun.
- *Seborrheic keratosis* with irregularly shaped borders and a scaly surface often occurs on the face, shoulders, and trunk. These benign lesions begin as yellowish to tan and progress to a dark brown or black.
- *Vitiligo* tends to increase with age and is thought to result from an autoimmune response.
- Cutaneous tags are most commonly seen in the neck and axillary regions. These skin lesions vary in size and are soft, often flesh-colored, and pedicled.
- Visible, bright red, fine, dilated blood vessels (*telangiectasias*) commonly occur as a result of the thinning of the dermis and the loss of support for the blood vessel walls.
- *Actinic keratoses* may appear at about age 50, often on the face, ears, backs of the hands, and arms. They may become malignant if untreated.

The Hair

- There may be loss of scalp, pubic, and axillary hair.
- Hairs of the eyebrows, ears, and nostrils become bristle-like and coarse.

The Nails

- The nails grow more slowly and thicken.
- Longitudinal bands commonly develop, and the nails tend to split.
- Bands across the nails may indicate protein deficiency; white spots, zinc deficiency; and spoon-shaped nails, iron deficiency.
- Toenail fungus is more common and difficult to eliminate (although not dangerous to health).

The Eyes and Vision

- Visual acuity decreases as the lens of the eye ages and becomes more opaque and loses elasticity.
- The ability of the iris to accommodate to darkness and dim light diminishes.
- Peripheral vision diminishes.
- The adaptation to light (glare) and dark decreases.
- Accommodation to far objects often improves, but accommodation to near objects decreases.
- Color vision declines; older people are less able to perceive purple colors and to discriminate pastel colors.
- Many older people wear corrective lenses; they are most likely to have hyperopia. Visual changes are due to loss of elasticity (presbyopia) and transparency of the lens.
- The skin around the orbit of the eye may darken.
- The eyeball may appear sunken because of the decrease in orbital fat.
- Skinfolds of the upper lids may seem more prominent, and the lower lids may sag.
- The eyes may appear dry and lusterless because of the decrease in tear production from the lacrimal glands.
- *Arcus senilis* appears around part or all of the cornea. It results from an accumulation of a lipid substance on the cornea. The cornea tends to cloud with age.
- The iris may appear pale with brown discolorations as a result of pigment degeneration.
- The conjunctiva of the eye may appear paler than that of younger adults and may take on a slightly yellow appearance because of the deposition of fat.
- Pupil reaction to light and accommodation is normally symmetric but may be less brisk.
- The pupils can appear smaller in size, unequal, and irregular in shape because of sclerotic changes in the iris.

The Ears and Hearing

- The skin of the ear may appear dry and be less resilient because of the loss of connective tissue.
- Increased coarse and wirelike hair growth occurs along the helix, antihelix, and tragus.
- The pinna increases in both width and length, and the earlobe elongates.
- Earwax is drier.
- The tympanic membrane is more translucent and less flexible. The intensity of the light reflex may diminish slightly.
- Sensorineural hearing loss occurs.
- Generalized hearing loss (presbycusis) occurs in all frequencies, although the first symptom is the loss of high-frequency sounds: the *f, s, sh,* and *ph* sounds. To such persons, conversation can be distorted and result in what appears to be inappropriate or confused behavior.

The Nose and Sinuses

- The sense of smell markedly diminishes because of a decrease in the number of olfactory nerve fibers and atrophy of the remaining fibers. Older adults are less able to identify and discriminate odors.
- Nosebleeds may result from hypertensive disease or other arterial vessel changes.

The Mouth

- The oral mucosa may be drier than that of younger persons because of decreased salivary gland activity. Decreased salivation occurs only in older adults taking prescribed medications such as antidepressants, antihistamines, decongestants, diuretics, antihypertensives, tranquilizers, antispasmodics, and antineoplastics. Extreme dryness is associated with dehydration.
- Some receding of the gums occurs, giving an appearance of increased toothiness.

- The gums may develop a brownish pigmentation, especially in blacks.
- Taste sensations diminish. Sweet and salty tastes are lost first. Older adults may add more salt and sugar to food than they did when they were younger. Diminished taste sensation is due to atrophy of the taste buds and a decreased sense of smell. It indicates diminished function of the fifth and seventh cranial nerves.
- Tiny purple or bluish-black swollen areas (varicosities) under the tongue, known as *caviar spots,* are not uncommon.
- The teeth may show signs of staining, erosion, chipping, and abrasions due to loss of dentin. Tooth loss occurs as a result of dental disease but is preventable with good dental hygiene.
- The gag reflex may be slightly sluggish.

The Thorax and Lungs

- The thoracic curvature may be accentuated (kyphosis) because of osteoporosis and changes in cartilage, resulting in collapse of the vertebrae.
- Kyphosis and osteoporosis alter the size of the chest cavity as the ribs move downward and forward.
- The anteroposterior diameter of the chest widens, giving a barrel-chested appearance.
- Breathing rate and rhythm are unchanged at rest; the rate normally increases with exercise but may take longer to return to the preexercise rate.
- Inspiratory muscles become less powerful, and the inspiration reserve volume decreases. A decrease in depth of respiration is therefore apparent.
- Expiration may require the use of accessory muscles. The expiratory reserve volume significantly increases because of the increased amount of air remaining in the lungs at the end of a normal breath.
- Deflation of the lung is incomplete.

- Small airways lose their cartilaginous support and elastic recoil; as a result, they tend to close, particularly in basal or dependent portions of the lung.
- Elastic tissue of the alveoli loses its stretchability and changes to fibrous tissue. Exertional capacity decreases.
- Cilia in the airways decrease in number and are less effective in removing mucus; older adults are therefore at greater risk for pulmonary infections.

The Cardiovascular and Peripheral Vascular Systems

- Cardiac output and strength of contraction decrease, thus lessening the older adult's activity tolerance.
- The heart rate returns to its resting rate more slowly after exertion than it did when the individual was younger.
- S_4 heart sound is considered normal in older adults.
- Extra systoles (premature ventricular contractions) commonly occur. Ten or more extra systoles per minute are considered abnormal.
- Sudden emotional and physical stresses may result in cardiac arrhythmias and heart failure.
- The overall effectiveness of blood vessels decreases as smooth muscle cells are replaced by connective tissue. The lower extremities are more likely to show signs of arterial and venous impairment because of the more distal and dependent position.
- Proximal arteries become thinner and dilate.
- Peripheral arteries become thicker and dilate less effectively because of arteriosclerotic changes in the vessel walls.
- Blood vessels lengthen and become more tortuous and prominent. Varicosities occur more frequently.
- In some instances, arteries may be palpated more easily because of the loss of supportive surrounding tissues. Often, however, the most distal pulses of the lower extremities are more difficult to palpate because of decreased arterial perfusion.

- Systolic and diastolic blood pressures increase, but the increase in the systolic pressure is greater. As a result, the pulse pressure widens. Any client with a blood pressure reading above 140/90 should be referred for follow-up assessments.
- Peripheral edema is frequently observed and is most commonly the result of chronic venous insufficiency or low protein levels in the blood (hypoproteinemia).

The Abdomen
The Breasts and Axillae

- In the postmenopausal female, breasts change in shape and often appear pendulous or flaccid; they lack the firmness they had in younger years.
- The presence of breast lesions may be detected more readily because of the decrease in connective tissue.
- General breast size remains the same. Although glandular tissue atrophies, the amount of fat in breasts (predominantly in the lower quadrants) increases in most women.
- The rounded abdomens of older adults are due to an increase in adipose tissue and a decrease in muscle tone.
- The abdominal wall is slacker and thinner, making palpation easier and more accurate than in younger clients. Muscle wasting and loss of fibroconnective tissue occur.
- The pain threshold in older adults is often higher; major abdominal problems such as appendicitis or other acute emergencies may therefore go undetected.
- Gastrointestinal pain needs to be differentiated from cardiac pain. Gastrointestinal pain may be located in the chest or abdomen, whereas cardiac pain is usually located in the chest. Factors aggravating gastrointestinal pain are usually related to either ingestion or lack of food intake; gastrointestinal pain is usually relieved by antacids, food, or assuming an upright position. Common factors that can aggravate cardiac pain are activity or anxiety; rest or nitroglycerin relieves cardiac pain.

- Stool passes through the intestines at a slower rate in older adults, and the perception of stimuli that produce the urge to defecate often diminishes.
- Fecal incontinence may occur in confused or neurologically impaired older adults.
- The incidence of colon cancer is higher among older adults than younger adults. Symptoms include a change in bowel function, rectal bleeding, and weight loss. Changes in bowel function, however, are associated with many factors, such as diet, exercise, and medications.
- Decreased absorption of oral medications often occurs with aging.
- In the liver, impaired metabolism of some drugs may occur with aging.

The Musculoskeletal System

- Muscle mass decreases progressively with age, although wide variations exist among different individuals.
- The decrease in speed, strength, resistance to fatigue, reaction time, and coordination in older adults is due to a decrease in nerve conduction and muscle tone.
- The bones become more fragile, and osteoporosis leads to a loss of total bone mass. As a result, older adults are predisposed to fractures and compressed vertebrae.
- In most older adults, osteoarthritic changes in the joints can be observed.

The Neurologic System

- A full neurologic assessment can be lengthy. Conduct in several sessions if indicated and cease the tests if the client is noticeably fatigued.
- A decline in mental status is not a normal result of aging. Changes are more the result of physical or psychological disorders (e.g., fever, fluid and electrolyte imbalances). Acute, abrupt-onset mental status changes are usually caused by delirium. These

changes are often reversible with treatment. Chronic subtle insidious mental health changes are usually caused by dementia and are usually irreversible.

- Intelligence and learning ability are unaltered with age. Many factors, however, inhibit learning (e.g., anxiety, illness, pain, cultural barrier).
- Short-term memory is often less efficient. Long-term memory is usually unaltered.
- Because old age is often associated with loss of support persons, depression is a common disorder. Mood changes, weight loss, anorexia, constipation, and early-morning awakening may manifest it.
- The stress of being in unfamiliar situations can cause confusion in older adults.
- As a person ages, reflex responses may become less intense.
- Because older adults tire more easily than younger clients, a total neurologic assessment is often done at a different time than the other parts of the physical assessment.
- Although there is a progressive decrease in the number of functioning neurons in the central nervous system and in the sense organs, the older adult usually functions well because of the abundant reserves in the number of brain cells.
- Impulse transmission and reaction to stimuli are slower.
- Many older adults have some impairment of hearing, vision, smell, temperature and pain sensation, memory, and mental endurance.
- Coordination changes, including a reduced speed of fine finger movements. Standing balance remains intact, and Romberg's test remains negative.
- Reflex responses may slightly increase or decrease. Many show loss of Achilles reflex, and the plantar reflex may be difficult to elicit.

- When testing sensory function, give older adults time to respond. Normally, older adults have unaltered perception of light touch and superficial pain, decreased perception of deep pain, and decreased perception of temperature stimuli. Many also reveal a decrease or absence of position sense in the large toes.

The Genitals

- Labia become atrophied and flatten.
- The clitoris is a common site for cancerous lesions.
- The vulva atrophies as a result of a reduction in vascularity, elasticity, adipose tissue, and estrogen levels. Because the vulva is more fragile, it is more easily irritated.
- The vaginal environment becomes drier and more alkaline, resulting in an alteration of the type of flora present and a predisposition to vaginitis. Dyspareunia (difficult or painful coitus) is also a common occurrence.
- The cervix and uterus decrease in size.
- The fallopian tubes and ovaries atrophy.
- Ovulation and estrogen production cease.
- Prolapse of the uterus can occur, especially in those who have had multiple pregnancies.
- The penis decreases in size with age; the size and firmness of the testes decrease.
- Testosterone is produced in smaller amounts.
- More time and direct physical stimulation are required for an older man to achieve an erection, but he can maintain the erection for a longer period before ejaculation than he could at a younger age.
- Seminal fluid is reduced in amount and viscosity.
- Urinary frequency, nocturia, dribbling, and problems with beginning and ending the stream are usually the result of prostatic enlargement.

E. Nursing Diagnoses

Formulating Diagnostic Statements

The basic two-part statement includes the following:

1. *Problem (P):* statement of the client's response (NANDA label)
2. *Etiology (E):* factors contributing to or probable causes of the responses

Sample Two-Part Diagnostic Statements

Problem	Related to	Etiology
Constipation	Related to	Prolonged laxative use
Severe anxiety	Related to	Threat to physiologic integrity: possible cancer diagnosis

The basic three-part nursing diagnosis statement is called the *PES format* and includes the following:

1. *Problem (P):* statement of the client's response (NANDA label)
2. *Etiology (E):* factors contributing to or probable causes of the response
3. *Signs and symptoms (S):* defining characteristics manifested by the client

Sample Three-Part Diagnostic Statement

Problem	Related to	Etiology	As Manifested by	Signs and Symptoms
Situational low self-esteem	Related to (r/t)	Feelings of rejection by husband	As manifested by (a.m.b.)	Hypersensitivity to criticism; states "I don't know if I can manage by myself" and rejects positive feedback

2009-2011 NANDA-Approved Nursing Diagnoses

Activity Intolerance

Activity Intolerance, Risk for

Activity Planning, Ineffective

Airway Clearance, Ineffective

Anxiety

Anxiety, Death

Aspiration, Risk for

Attachment, Risk for Impaired

Autonomic Dysreflexia

Autonomic Dysreflexia, Risk for

Bleeding, Risk for

Blood Glucose Level, Risk for Unstable

Body Image, Disturbed

Body Temperature: Imbalanced, Risk for

Bowel Incontinence

Breastfeeding, Effective

Breastfeeding, Ineffective

Breastfeeding, Interrupted

Breathing Pattern, Ineffective

Cardiac Output, Decreased
Caregiver Role Strain
Caregiver Role Strain, Risk for
Childbearing Process, Readiness for Enhanced
Comfort, Impaired
Comfort, Readiness for Enhanced
Communication, Impaired Verbal
Communication, Readiness for Enhanced
Confusion, Acute
Confusion, Acute, Risk for
Confusion, Chronic
Constipation
Constipation, Perceived
Constipation, Risk for
Contamination
Contamination, Risk for
Coping: Community, Ineffective
Coping: Community, Readiness for Enhanced
Coping, Defensive
Coping: Family, Compromised
Coping: Family, Disabled
Coping: Family, Readiness for Enhanced
Coping, Readiness for Enhanced
Coping, Ineffective
Decisional Conflict
Decision-Making, Readiness for Enhanced
Denial, Ineffective
Dentition, Impaired
Development: Delayed, Risk for
Diarrhea
Disuse Syndrome, Risk for
Diversional Activity, Deficient

Electrolyte Imbalance, Risk for
Energy Field, Disturbed
Environmental Interpretation Syndrome, Impaired
Failure to Thrive, Adult
Falls, Risk for
Family Processes, Dysfunctional
Family Processes, Interrupted
Family Processes, Readiness for Enhanced
Fatigue
Fear
Fluid Balance, Readiness for Enhanced
Fluid Volume, Deficient
Fluid Volume, Deficient, Risk for
Fluid Volume, Excess
Fluid Volume, Imbalanced, Risk for
Gas Exchange, Impaired
Gastrointestinal Motility, Dysfunctional
Gastrointestinal Motility, Dysfunctional, Risk for
Grieving
Grieving, Complicated
Grieving, Risk for Complicated
Growth, Disproportionate, Risk for
Growth and Development, Delayed
Health Behavior, Risk-Prone
Health Maintenance, Ineffective
Health Management, Ineffective Self
Health Management, Readiness for Enhanced Self
Health-Seeking Behaviors (Specify)
Home Maintenance, Impaired
Hope, Readiness for Enhanced
Hopelessness
Human Dignity, Risk for Compromised

Hyperthermia
Hypothermia
Immunization Status, Readiness for Enhanced
Infant Behavior, Disorganized
Infant Behavior: Disorganized, Risk for
Infant Behavior: Organized, Readiness for Enhanced
Infant Feeding Pattern, Ineffective
Infection, Risk for
Injury, Risk for
Insomnia
Intracranial Adaptive Capacity, Decreased
Jaundice, Neonatal
Knowledge, Deficient
Knowledge, Readiness for Enhanced
Latex Allergy Response
Latex Allergy Response, Risk for
Liver Function, Impaired, Risk for
Loneliness, Risk for
Maternal/Fetal Dyad, Risk for Disturbed
Memory, Impaired
Mobility: Bed, Impaired
Mobility: Physical, Impaired
Mobility: Wheelchair, Impaired
Moral Distress
Nausea
Neglect, Self
Neglect, Unilateral
Neurovascular Dysfunction: Peripheral, Risk for
Noncompliance (Specify)
Nutrition, Imbalanced: Less than Body Requirements

Nutrition, Imbalanced: More than Body Requirements

Nutrition, Imbalanced: More than Body Requirements, Risk for

Nutrition, Readiness for Enhanced

Oral Mucous Membrane, Impaired

Pain, Acute

Pain, Chronic

Parenting, Impaired

Parenting, Readiness for Enhanced

Parenting, Risk for Impaired

Perfusion, Decreased Cardiac Tissue, Risk for

Perfusion, Ineffective Cerebral Tissue, Risk for

Perfusion, Ineffective Gastrointestinal, Risk for

Perfusion, Ineffective Peripheral Tissue

Perfusion, Ineffective Renal, Risk for

Perioperative Positioning Injury, Risk for

Personal Identity, Disturbed

Poisoning, Risk for

Post-Trauma Syndrome

Post-Trauma Syndrome, Risk for

Power, Readiness for Enhanced

Powerlessness

Powerlessness, Risk for

Protection, Ineffective

Rape-Trauma Syndrome

Relationship, Readiness for Enhanced

Religiosity, Impaired

Religiosity, Readiness for Enhanced

Religiosity, Risk for Impaired

Relocation Stress Syndrome

Relocation Stress Syndrome, Risk for

Resilience, Risk for Compromised

Resilience, Impaired Individual

Resilience, Readiness for Enhanced

Role Conflict, Parental

Role Performance, Ineffective

Sedentary Lifestyle

Self-Care, Readiness for Enhanced

Self-Care Deficit: Bathing

Self-Care Deficit: Dressing

Self-Care Deficit: Feeding

Self-Care Deficit: Toileting

Self-Concept, Readiness for Enhanced

Self-Esteem, Chronic Low

Self-Esteem, Situational Low

Self-Esteem, Risk for Situational Low

Self-Mutilation

Self-Mutilation, Risk for

Sensory Perception, Disturbed (Specify: Auditory, Gustatory, Kinesthetic, Olfactory, Tactile, Visual)

Sexual Dysfunction

Sexuality Pattern, Ineffective

Shock, Risk for

Skin Integrity, Impaired

Skin Integrity, Risk for Impaired

Sleep Deprivation

Sleep, Readiness for Enhanced

Sleep Pattern, Disturbed

Social Interaction, Impaired

Social Isolation

Sorrow, Chronic

Spiritual Distress

Spiritual Distress, Risk for
Spiritual Well-Being, Readiness for Enhanced
Spontaneous Ventilation, Impaired
Stress Overload
Sudden Infant Death Syndrome, Risk for
Suffocation, Risk for
Suicide, Risk for
Surgical Recovery, Delayed
Swallowing, Impaired
Therapeutic Regimen Management: Ineffective Family
Thermoregulation, Ineffective
Tissue Integrity, Impaired
Transfer Ability, Impaired
Trauma, Risk for
Trauma, Vascular, Risk for
Urinary Elimination, Impaired
Urinary Elimination, Readiness for Enhanced
Urinary Incontinence, Functional
Urinary Incontinence, Overflow
Urinary Incontinence, Reflex
Urinary Incontinence, Stress
Urinary Incontinence, Urge
Urinary Retention
Ventilatory Weaning Response, Dysfunctional
Violence: Other-Directed, Risk for
Violence: Self-Directed, Risk for
Walking, Impaired
Wandering

Source: NANDA International (2009). *Nursing Diagnoses: Definitions and Classification 2009–2011.* Oxford, UK: Wiley-Blackwell. Used with permission.

UNIT 3

PLANNING AND IMPLEMENTATION

A. Safety Guidelines
   1. Guidelines Related to Body Mechanics and Safe Client Handling and Movement
   2. Preventing Falls in Health Care Agencies
   3. Adult Home Hazard Appraisal
   4. Steps to Follow in the Event of Fire
B. Clinical Guidelines
   1. Fluid and Electrolyte Balance
   2. Individualizing Care for Clients with Pain
   3. Respiratory Function
   4. Tube Feedings
   5. Urinary Elimination
   6. Fecal Elimination
   7. Pressure Areas
   8. Healing Wounds
   9. Postoperative Period
C. Teaching and Learning Guidelines
D. Medications
   1. Methods of Calculating Dosages
   2. Injection Techniques

A. Safety Guidelines

To be a safe practitioner, you must know your limitations, know how and when to seek information, and stay current in your field. As health care advances, techniques are modified. Attend classes, read the literature, and become familiar with your responsibilities as set forth by your agency. For example, cardiopulmonary resuscitation certification is required by most health care facilities; do not allow your certification to lapse.

Many health care agencies also have specific guidelines or procedures to follow in the event of an emergency, such as fire. Familiarize yourself with this information each time you go to a new facility. On each unit, make sure you know the location of the exit doors, the stairs, the crash cart, and the fire extinguishers. The first rule of safety is preparedness.

Know your resources. Find out where on the unit the procedure manuals are kept. If you are unfamiliar with a procedure, look it up. Knowing your resources also means knowing to whom you can go with questions or whom to seek out for advice. Your clinical instructor is one of your best safety resources. This person knows your level of knowledge, your clinical skill level, and your anxiety level. If you have concerns, talk them out with your instructor. Never perform skills that you are unsure of; always review the skill and seek assistance if you feel uncertain. See Chapter 32 of *Fundamentals of Nursing* for a thorough discussion of safety guidelines.

Investigate the availability of resource manuals. Does your unit have a current drug handbook? Be familiar with all medications that you administer: Carry a drug handbook, or consult a unit handbook before administering medications. If you still have questions, go to your instructor for help. Be aware that the pharmacy staff is there to help you; pharmacists are particularly helpful for answering questions about new drugs, discussing drug–drug interactions, and planning medication schedules for clients.

Do not take unnecessary risks. Follow standard precautions to protect yourself from bloodborne pathogens. See pages 155 to 163 for a quick reference on standard precautions. To provide safe care, you must also use good body mechanics. Even when using good body mechanics, the average nurse should not lift more than 35 pounds and only under very controlled circumstances. Client-handling tasks (e.g., transfers) are performed at high risk for the nurse. There is no safe way to perform manual client handling. The development of assistive client handling equipment and devices (e.g., floor-based and ceiling lifts, stand-to-assist lifts) have made "manual" and "solo" client handling unnecessary. Summaries of body mechanics guidelines and other safety guidelines are provided next.

1. Guidelines Related to Body Mechanics and Safe Client Handling and Movement

Body Mechanics

- Start any body movement with proper alignment.
- Stand as close as possible to the object to be moved.
- Avoid stretching, reaching, and twisting, which may place the line of gravity outside your base of support.
- Before moving an object, widen your stance and flex your knees, hips, and ankles.
- Adjust the working area to waist level, and keep your body close to the area.
- Put the bed at the correct height (waist level when providing care; hip level when moving a client).
- To prevent stretching and reaching, elevate adjustable beds and overbed tables, or lower the side rails of beds.

- When pushing an object, enlarge your base of support by moving your front foot forward.
- When pulling an object, enlarge your base of support either by moving the rear leg back (if you are facing the object) or by moving the front foot forward (if you are facing away from the object).
- Before moving objects, contract your gluteal, abdominal, leg, and arm muscles to prepare them for action.
- Use your gluteal and leg muscles rather than the sacrospinal muscles of your back to exert an upward thrust.
- Distribute the workload between both arms and legs to prevent back strain.
- Always face the direction of the movement to prevent twisting of the spine and ineffective use of major muscle groups.
- When moving or carrying objects, hold them as close as possible to your center of gravity.
- Use arms as levers when possible to increase lifting power.
- Use your own body weight to counteract the weight of the object you are moving. For example, lean forward when pushing an object, and rock your body weight backward when pulling an object or client toward you.
- Avoid working against gravity.
- Lower the head of the client's bed before moving the client up in bed.

Safe Client Handling and Movement

- Assess the following before performing client handling and movement:
  - Client's Level of Assistance: Independent, Partial Assist or Dependent
  - Client's Weight-Bearing Ability: Full, Partial or None
  - Client's Bilateral Upper-Extremity Strength: Yes or No

- Client's Level of Participation and Comprehension: Cooperative, Unpredictable, or Varies
- Client's weight and height
- Are there conditions that can affect transfer/repositioning of client? (e.g., hip/knee/shoulder replacements, history of falls, respiratory/cardiac compromise, paralysis)
- Appropriate Lift/Transfer Devices Needed

- Obtain the assistance of other people or use mechanical devices if the maximum weight for the manual lift exceeds 35 pounds.
- Plan the move or transfer carefully. Free the surrounding area of obstacles.
- Encourage clients to assist as much as possible.
- Use arms as levers whenever possible to increase lifting power.

2. Preventing Falls in Health Care Agencies

- Orient clients upon admission to their surroundings, and explain the call system.
- Carefully assess the client's ability to ambulate and transfer; provide walking aids and assistance as required.
- Closely supervise the clients at risk for falls during the first few days, especially at night.
- Encourage the client to use the call bell to request assistance; ensure that the bell is within reach.
- Place bedside tables and overbed tables near the bed or chair so that clients do not overreach and consequently lose their balance.
- Always keep hospital beds in the low position when not providing care so that clients can move into or out of bed easily.
- Encourage clients to use grab bars mounted in toilet and bathing areas and railings along corridors.

- Make sure nonskid bath mats are available in tubs and showers.
- Encourage the client to wear nonskid footwear.
- Keep the environment tidy, especially keep light cords from underfoot and furniture out of the way.
- Reduce poor lighting and glare, which causes clients to squint.
- Use individualized interventions (e.g., alarm sensitive to client position) rather than side rails for confused clients.
- Use mechanical or electronic ceiling lifts to transfer dependent clients.

3. Adult Home Hazard Appraisal

- *Walkways and stairways (inside and outside).* Note uneven sidewalks or paths, broken or loose steps, absence of handrails or placement on only one side of stairways, insecure handrails, congested hallways or other traffic areas, and adequacy of lighting at night.
- *Floors.* Note uneven and highly polished or slippery floors and any unanchored rugs or mats.
- *Furniture.* Note hazardous placement of furniture with sharp corners. Note chairs or stools that are too low to get into and out of or that provide inadequate support.
- *Bathroom(s).* Note the presence of grab bars around tubs and toilets, nonslip surfaces in tubs and shower stalls, adequacy of lighting for medicine cabinet, and need for raised toilet seat or bath chair in tub or shower.
- *Kitchen.* Note pilot lights (gas stove) in need of repair, inaccessible storage areas, and hazardous furniture. Check for presence of operational smoke detector.
- *Bedrooms.* Note adequacy of lighting, in particular the availability of night-lights and accessibility of light switches. Assess floors and furniture as previously. Note access to bathroom.
- *Electrical.* Note unanchored and/or frayed electrical cords, overloaded outlets, and any outlets near water.

- *Fire protection.* Note the presence or absence of a fire extinguisher and fire escape plan, improper storage of combustibles (e.g., gasoline) or corrosives [e.g., rust remover (phosphoric acid)], and accessibility of emergency telephone numbers (fire, police).
- *Toxic substances.* Note appropriate storage of medicines or toxic substances such as cleaning solutions. Note medications kept beyond date of expiration and improperly labeled cleaning solutions.

4. Steps to Follow in the Event of Fire

In health care agencies, fire is particularly hazardous when people are incapacitated and unable to leave the building without assistance. This incapacity makes it extremely important for nurses to be aware of the fire safety regulations and fire prevention practices of the agencies in which they work. When smoke or fire is detected, two mnemonics can help the nurse remember the steps to follow. First is the RACE protocol:

1. Rescue: If the area is safe to enter, protect and evacuate clients who are in immediate danger.
2. Activate: Pull the fire alarm and report the fire details and location to the hospital's fire emergency extension.
3. Confine: Contain the fire by closing the doors to all rooms and the fire doors at each entrance to the unit.
4. Extinguish: Extinguish the fire. Use the appropriate type of fire extinguisher (see the PASS mnemonic).

Extinguishing the fire requires knowledge of three categories of fire, classified according to the type of material that is burning:

Class A: Paper, wood, upholstery, rags, ordinary rubbish

Class B: Flammable liquids and gases

Class C: Electrical

The right type of extinguisher must be used to fight the fire. Extinguishers have picture symbols showing the type of fire for which they are to be used. Directions for use are also attached. The nurse follows the mnemonic PASS when using a fire extinguisher:

Pull out the extinguisher's safety pin.

Aim the hose at the base of the fire.

Squeeze the handle to discharge the material onto the fire.

Sweep the hose from side to side across the base of the fire until extinguished.

B. Clinical Guidelines

1. Fluid and Electrolyte Balance

Assess to Determine

- The usual amount and type of fluids ingested each day
- Foods rich in protein, sodium, potassium, and calcium eaten each day
- Any recent changes in food or fluid intake and reason (e.g., presence of nausea, pain, anorexia, or dysphagia)
- Any recent changes in frequency or amount of urine output
- Major losses of body fluid through vomiting, diarrhea, excessive perspiration, or other route (e.g., drainage from gastrointestinal function, ileostomy, colostomy, or burn sites)
- History of any long-term or recent disease processes that might disrupt fluid, electrolyte, and acid–base balance: kidney disease, heart disease, high blood pressure, diabetes mellitus, diabetes insipidus, thyroid or parathyroid disorders, asthma, emphysema, severe trauma, or other chronic disease states (e.g., cancer, colitis, ileitis)
- Medication therapy that could affect fluid and electrolyte balance: diuretics, steroids, potassium supplements, or aldosterone inhibitor agents
- Recent treatments that could affect fluid and electrolyte balance, such as dialysis, total parenteral nutrition, tube drainage (e.g., nasogastric or intestinal suction), or tube feedings

Assess the Client for

- Signs that indicate insufficient hydration: excessive thirst, dry skin and mucous membranes, concentrated urine, reduced urine output, poor tissue turgor, depressed periorbital spaces
- Signs indicating excessive hydration: swollen ankles, difficulty breathing, sudden weight gain, ascites, moist crackles (rales) in lungs
- Signs that might indicate an electrolyte or acid–base imbalance: loss of mental alertness; disorientation; faintness; muscle weakness, twitching, cramps, fatigue, pain, or spasm; abnormal sensations (e.g., burning, prickling, tingling); abdominal cramps or distention; heart palpitations

Obtain Clinical Measurements

- *Baseline and daily weight.* Rapid losses or gains of 5% or more of total body weight indicate moderate to severe fluid volume deficit or excess.
- *Vital signs. Body temperature:* An increased body temperature may indicate hypernatremic dehydration; a decreased body temperature may result from hypovolemia. *Pulse rate*: An increased pulse rate and a weak, thready pulse may occur with fluid volume deficit or potassium excess. *Respiration*: An increased rate with adventitious sounds may indicate a fluid volume excess. An increased rate and depth of respiration may cause carbonic acid deficit (respiratory alkalosis); shallow respirations may create a carbonic acid excess (respiratory acidosis). Either may be a compensatory mechanism for metabolic acid–base imbalances. *Blood pressure*: An elevated systolic blood pressure may indicate a fluid volume excess; a sudden decreased systolic pressure exceeding 10 mm Hg usually indicates a fluid volume deficit.
- Twenty-four–hour fluid intake and output.

Review Results of Laboratory Tests

- Serum electrolyte levels
- Hematocrit

- Urine specific gravity
- Arterial blood gases

Identify Clients at Risk for Fluid and Electrolyte Imbalances

- Postoperative clients
- Clients with severe trauma or burns
- Clients with chronic diseases, such as heart failure, diabetes, chronic obstructive lung disease, and cancer
- Clients who are permitted nothing by mouth
- Clients with intravenous infusions
- Clients with retention catheters and urinary drainage systems
- Clients with special drainages or suctions, such as a nasogastric suction
- Clients receiving diuretics
- Clients experiencing excessive fluid losses and requiring increased intake
- Clients who retain fluids
- Clients with fluid restrictions
- Older adults who may not be taking in the fluids they need
- Clients unable to respond to the thirst sensation (e.g., comatose clients)
- Clients receiving electrolyte therapy (e.g., potassium supplements)
- Clients unable to communicate desire for fluid (e.g., very young and very old clients)
- Clients with very high or very low total body water

Monitoring Fluid Intake and Output

- To assess fluid balance, determine the client's intake and output, and observe the client for signs of dehydration or overhydration.
- Monitor intake and output for all clients (a) whose oral fluid intake is insufficient, (b) who are experiencing

excessive fluid loss via normal or abnormal routes, (c) who are retaining fluid, or (d) who are taking medications that alter fluid output.

- Weigh clients who are retaining fluid or receiving diuretics daily.

Facilitating Normal or Increased Fluid Intake

- Explain to the client the reason for the required intake and the specific amount needed. This gives the client a rationale for the requirement and thus promotes compliance.
- Establish a 24-hour plan for ingesting the fluids. Generally, half of the total volume is ingested during the day shift, and the other half is divided between the evening and night shifts, with the majority ingested during the evening shift. For example, if 2500 mL is to be ingested in 24 hours, the plan may specify that 1500 mL be ingested in the 7-to-3 shift, 700 mL in the 3-to-11 shift, and 300 mL in the 11-to-7 shift. To prevent the need to urinate during sleeping hours, clients should avoid ingesting large amounts of fluid before bedtime.
- Set short-term outcomes that the client can realistically meet. For example, the client might ingest a glass of fluid every hour while awake or a pitcher of water by noon.
- Identify fluids the client likes, and make available a variety of those items. Examples may include fruit juices, tea, coffee, and milk (if allowed).
- Help clients to select foods that tend to become liquid at room temperature (e.g., gelatin, ice cream, sherbert, custard), if these are allowed.
- For clients who are confined to bed, supply appropriate cups, glasses, and straws to facilitate appropriate fluid intake. Keep the fluids within easy reach.
- Make sure fluids are served at the appropriate temperature: hot fluids hot, and cold fluids iced and cold.
- Encourage clients to participate in maintaining the fluid intake record, when possible. This helps them determine whether they are achieving preestablished goals.

- Be alert for the cultural implications of food and fluids. Some cultures may restrict certain foods and fluids and view others as having healing properties.

Helping Clients Restrict Fluid Intake

- Explain the reason for the restricted intake and how much and what types of fluids are permitted orally. Many clients need to be informed that ice chips, gelatin, and ice cream, for example, are considered fluid.
- Help the client decide how to allocate the total amount of fluid allowed: how much to take with each meal, between meals, before bedtime, and with medications. Generally, half of the total volume is scheduled during the day shift, when the client is most active, receives two meals, and, often, most oral medications. A large part of the remainder is scheduled for the evening shift to permit the client to take fluids with meals and during evening visits.
- Identify fluids the client likes, and make sure that these are provided, unless contraindicated. A client who is allowed only 200 mL of fluid for breakfast, for example, should receive the type of fluid the client favors.
- Set short-term goals that make the fluid restriction more tolerable. For example, schedule a specified amount of fluid at 1- or 2-hour intervals between meals. Some clients may prefer fluids between meals only, because the food provided at mealtime may help relieve feelings of thirst.
- Provide the client with small fluid containers that make the container appear to contain more fluid than it actually does.
- Periodically offer the client ice chips as an alternative to water. Ice chips occupy twice the volume of an equal amount of water.
- Help clients rinse their mouths with water if they can do so without swallowing the fluid.
- Ensure meticulous oral care.

- Instruct the client to avoid ingesting or chewing salty or sweet foods (hard candy or gum) because these foods tend to produce thirst. Sugarless gum may be an alternative for some clients.
- Encourage the client to participate in maintaining the fluid intake record, when possible.

Special Care for Older Adults

Fluid and Electrolyte Balance

Certain changes related to aging place the older adult at risk for serious problems with fluid and electrolyte imbalance, if homeostatic mechanisms are compromised. These changes include decreases in the following:

- Thirst sensation
- Ability of the kidneys to concentrate urine
- Intracellular fluid and total body water
- Response to body hormones that help regulate fluid and electrolytes

Other factors that may influence fluid and electrolyte balance in elders are the following:

- Increased use of diuretics for hypertension and heart disease
- Decrease in fluid and food intake, especially in clients with dementia or who are dependent on others to feed them and offer them fluids
- Preparations for certain diagnostic tests that have the client take nothing by mouth for long periods of time or cause diarrhea from laxative preparations
- Clients with impaired renal function, such as older adult clients and/or those with diabetes
- Those having certain diagnostic procedures. (Dyes used for some procedures, such as arteriograms and cardiac catheterizations, may cause further renal problems. Always see that the client is well hydrated before, during, and after the procedure to help in diluting

and excreting the dye. If the client can take nothing by mouth for the procedure, the nurse should check with the primary care provider to see if intravenous fluids are needed.)

- Any condition that may tax the normal compensatory mechanisms, such as a fever, influenza, surgery, or heat exposure

These conditions increase the elder's risk for fluid and electrolyte imbalance. The change can happen quickly and become serious in a short time. Astute observations and quick actions by the nurse can help prevent serious consequences. A change in mental status may be the first symptom of impairment and must be further evaluated to determine the cause.

2. Individualizing Care for Clients with Pain

- Establish a trusting relationship. Convey your concern and acknowledge that you believe the client is experiencing pain. A trusting relationship encourages the client to express thoughts and feelings and enhances the effectiveness of planned pain therapies.
- Assess the source of the pain carefully. The source of the pain may not always be what is apparent. For example, the postoperative client who has had abdominal surgery may complain of pain related to a headache or other discomfort.
- Consider the client's ability and willingness to participate actively in pain-relief measures. Excessively fatigued or sedated clients or those who have altered levels of consciousness are less able to actively participate.
- Use a variety of pain relief measures. It is thought that using more than one measure has an additive effect in relieving pain. Two measures that should always be part of a pain relief plan are (a) establishing a trusting client–nurse relationship and (b) client teaching. Because a client's pain may vary throughout a 24-hour

period, different types of pain relief are often indicated during that time.

- Provide measures to relieve pain before it becomes severe. For example, it is better to provide an analgesic before pain is expected than to wait for the client to complain of pain, when a larger dose may be required.
- Use pain relief measures that the client believes are effective. It has been recognized that clients are often knowledgeable about measures that are effective in relieving their own pain. Therefore, incorporate the client's measures into a pain relief plan, unless they are harmful.
- Consider the client's willingness to participate actively in pain-relief measures.
- Base the choice of the pain-relief measure on the client's report of the severity of the pain. If a client reports mild pain, an analgesic such as aspirin may be indicated, whereas a client who reports severe pain may require a more potent relief measure.
- If a pain-relief measure proves to be ineffective, encourage the client to try it once or twice more before abandoning it. Anxiety may inhibit the effectiveness of a pain-relief measure, and some approaches, such as distraction strategies, require practice before they become effective.
- Maintain an unbiased attitude (open mind) about what may relieve the pain. New ways to relieve pain are continually being developed. It is not always possible to explain why a pain-relief measure works; however, you should support a measure unless it is harmful.
- Keep trying. Do *not* ignore a client because pain persists in spite of taking measures to relieve it. In these circumstances, reassess the pain, and consider other pain-relief measures.
- Prevent harm to the client. Pain therapy should not increase discomfort or harm the client.

- Educate the client and support persons about pain. Inform them about possible causes, precipitating and alleviating factors, and alternatives to drug therapy. Correct any misconceptions.

Cognitive-Behavioral Modalities

Whereas pharmacologic interventions aim at the pain itself, cognitive-behavioral modalities aim at reducing the resistance to pain, thus reducing suffering. Ample evidence from research is mounting to support the effectiveness of these modalities and their relative freedom from negative side effects. The goals of cognitive-behavioral interventions include providing comfort, altering psychological responses to reduce pain perception, and optimizing functioning. Selected cognitive-behavioral interventions include distraction, eliciting the relaxation response, repatterning unhelpful thinking, facilitating coping with emotions, and spiritual interventions.

- *Distraction.* Distraction draws the person's attention away from the pain and lessens the perception of pain. Distraction makes the person unaware of the pain only for the amount of time and to the extent that the distracting activity holds his or her "undivided" attention. Types of distraction include: Visual (reading or watching TV), Auditory (music), Tactile (slow, rhythmic breathing, needlework), and Intellectual (puzzles, card games, hobbies).
- *Eliciting the Relaxation Response.* The relaxation response decreases and counteracts the harmful effects of stress, including the effect it has on physical, cognitive, and emotional functioning. It involves a structured technique designed to focus the mind and relax muscle groups. Basic techniques with helpful scripts are available for common techniques including progressive relaxation, breath-focus relaxation, and meditation.
- *Repatterning Unhelpful Thinking.* Some people have strong self-doubts, unrealistic expectations (e.g., "I just

want someone to make the pain go away"), rumination (e.g., "I keep thinking about my pain and the person who did this to me"), helplessness (e.g., "I can't do anything"), and magnification (e.g., "My life is ruined, I'll never be a good parent because of my pain"). These cognitive patterns have been identified as important contributors to treatment failures, the intensification of pain, disability, and depression. Nurses can help by challenging the truthfulness and helpfulness of these thoughts, and replacing them with realistic and confidence-building ones that are particularly powerful predictors of more effective coping, better clinical outcomes, and improved quality of life.

- *Facilitating Coping.* Nurses can help by intervening with clients who are anxious, are sad, or express overly pessimistic or helpless points of view. Therapeutic communication with an emphasis on listening, providing encouragement, teaching self-management skills, sharing vicarious experiences, and persuading clients to act on their own behalf are strategies that enhance coping.
- *Selected Spiritual Interventions.* The spiritual dimension encompasses a person's innermost concerns and values, including the ascribed purpose, meaning, and driving force in the person's life. It may include rituals that help the individual become part of a community or feel a bond with the universe that is not necessarily religious in nature. For those who express their spirituality in a religious context, it is appropriate to offer prayer, intercessory prayer (being prayed for by others), or access to meaningful rituals. Scriptural readings may provide strength and comfort to clients in pain, and should be offered only when desired by the client. For some clients, a caring presence, attentive listening, and facilitating the process of acceptance can help reduce spiritual distress, whereas other clients benefit from manipulation of energy patterns (e.g., therapeutic touch).

Special Care for Older Adults

Pain Management

- Focus on the client's control in dealing with the pain.
- Spend time with the client and listen carefully.
- Clarify misconceptions. Encourage independence when possible.

Patient-Controlled Analgesia Pump

- Carefully monitor for drug side effects.
- Use cautiously for individuals with impaired pulmonary or renal function.
- Assess the client's cognitive and physical ability to use the client control button.

3. Respiratory Function

Assess to Determine

- *Current respiratory problems.* What recent changes has the client experienced in breathing pattern (e.g., shortness of breath, difficulty breathing, need to be in upright position to breathe, or rapid and shallow breathing)?
- *History of respiratory disease.* Has the client had colds, allergies, croup, asthma, tuberculosis, bronchitis, pneumonia, or emphysema? How frequently have these occurred? How long did they last? How were they treated?
- *Presence of a cough.* Is the cough productive or nonproductive? If productive, when is sputum produced? What are the amount, color, thickness, odor, and character of the sputum (e.g., thick, frothy, pink, rusty, or blood-tinged)?
- *Lifestyle.* Does the client smoke? If so, what (cigarettes, pipe, cigar) and how much? Does any member of the client's family smoke? Are there any occupational hazards (e.g., noxious fumes)?
- *Pain.* Does the client experience any pain associated with breathing or activity? Where is the pain located?

What words does the client use to describe the pain? How long does it last, and how does it affect breathing? What activities precede the pain?

- *Medication history.* Has the client taken or does the client take any over-the-counter or prescription medications for breathing? Which ones? What are the dosages, times taken, and effects on the client, including side effects?

Observe the Client's

- Breathing pattern (rate, rhythm, depth, and quality). Note any signs of hyperventilation or hypoventilation, tachypnea, or bradypnea.
- Ease or effort of breathing and posture assumed for breathing (e.g., orthopneic).
- Breath sounds audible without amplification (e.g., stridor, stertor, wheeze, bubbling).
- Chest movements (e.g., retractions, flail chest, or paradoxical breathing). Note the specific location of retractions: intercostal, substernal, suprasternal, or supraclavicular.
- Clinical signs of hypoxia or anoxia, such as increased pulse rate, rapid or deep respirations, cyanosis of the skin and nail beds, restlessness, anxiety, dizziness (vertigo), or faintness (syncope).
- The location of any surgical incision in relation to the muscles needed for breathing. An incision can impede appropriate lung expansion.

Palpate the Chest for

- Respiratory excursion
- Vocal (tactile) fremitus

Percuss the Chest for

- Diaphragmatic excursion
- Chest sounds (flatness, dullness, resonance, hyperresonance, tympany)

Auscultate the Lungs for

- Breath sounds (normal, adventitious, or absent). See the tables on pages 43 and 44.

Determine the Results of

- Sputum analysis
- Venous blood samples (e.g., complete blood count)
- Arterial blood samples (blood gases)
- Pulmonary function tests
- Pulse oximetry

Abnormal Breathing Patterns and Breath Sounds

Breathing Patterns

Rate

- Tachypnea—quick, shallow breaths
- Bradypnea—abnormally slow breathing
- Apnea—cessation of breathing

Volume

- Hyperventilation—overexpansion of the lungs characterized by rapid and deep breaths
- Hypoventilation—underexpansion of the lungs, characterized by shallow respirations

Rhythm

- Cheyne-Stokes breathing—rhythmic waxing and waning of respirations, from very deep to very shallow breathing and temporary apnea

Ease or Effort

- Dyspnea—difficult and labored breathing during which the individual has a persistent, unsatisfied need for air and feels distressed
- Orthopnea—ability to breathe only in upright sitting or standing positions

Breath Sounds

Audible without Amplification

- Stridor—a shrill, harsh sound heard during inspiration with laryngeal obstruction

- Stertor—snoring or sonorous respiration, usually due to a partial obstruction of the upper airway
- Wheeze—continuous, high-pitched musical squeak or whistling sound occurring on expiration and sometimes on inspiration when air moves through a narrowed or partially obstructed airway
- Bubbling—gurgling sounds heard as air passes through moist secretions in the respiratory tract

Audible by Stethoscope

- Crackles (rales)—dry or wet crackling sounds similar to the sound produced by rolling a lock of hair near the ear; generally heard on inspiration as air moves through accumulated moist secretions
- Gurgles (rhonchi)—coarse, leathery, or grating sound produced by the rubbing together of inflamed pleural tissues

Chest Movements

- Intercostal retraction—indrawing between the ribs
- Substernal retraction—indrawing beneath the breastbone
- Suprasternal retraction—indrawing above the clavicles

Secretions and Coughing

- Hemoptysis—the presence of blood in the sputum
- Productive cough—a cough accompanied by expectorated secretions
- Nonproductive cough—a dry, harsh cough without secretions

Oropharyngeal and Nasopharyngeal Suctioning

- Assess for clinical signs indicating the need for suctioning: restlessness; gurgling sounds during respiration; adventitious breath sounds when the chest is auscultated; change in mental status, skin color, rate and pattern of respirations, pulse rate, and rhythm. Reassess these after suctioning.
- Hyperventilate and hyperoxygenate the client before and after suctioning.

- In the unconscious client, prevent aspiration of sputum by positioning the person in the lateral position.
- Maintain sterility of the suction catheter, flushing solution, and gauzes used to wipe the catheter.
- Before the procedure, measure the correct length for catheter insertion.
- Moisten the catheter tip before insertion.
- Insert the catheter without applying suction. For tracheal suctioning, insert the catheter while the client inhales.
- Never force the catheter against an obstruction.
- Gently rotate the catheter while applying suction.
- Prevent or minimize hypoxia: Apply suction for no more than 15 seconds each time. Allow 20- to 30-second intervals between each suction, and limit suctioning to 5 minutes in total.
- Encourage deep breathing and coughing between suctions.
- Flush the catheter between suctions.
- Change suction collection bottles and tubing at least daily.

Special Care for Older Adults

- Older adults often have cardiac and/or pulmonary disease, thus increasing their susceptibility to hypoxemia related to suctioning. Watch closely for signs of hypoxemia. If noted, stop suctioning and hyperoxygenate.

4. Tube Feedings

Assess to Determine

- *Allergies to any food in the feeding.* Common ingredients in feedings include milk, sugar, water, eggs, and vegetable oil.
- *Bowel sounds before each feeding* (or every 4 to 8 hours for continuous feedings) to determine intestinal activity.

- *Abdominal distention at least daily.* Measure the client's abdominal girth at the umbilicus. A distended abdomen may indicate intolerance to a previous feeding.
- *Presence of regurgitation and feelings of fullness after feedings.*
- *Dumping syndrome.* Clients may experience nausea, vomiting, diarrhea, cramps, pallor, sweating, heart palpitations, increased pulse rate, and fainting after a feeding. Dumping syndrome results when hypertonic foods and liquids suddenly distend the jejunum. Smaller, more frequent feedings, and slower feedings may relieve dumping.
- *Presence of diarrhea, constipation, or flatulence.* The lack of bulk in liquid feedings may cause constipation. The presence of concentrated ingredients may cause diarrhea and flatulence.
- *Hydration status.* Measure the client's fluid intake and output, and note complaints of thirst. Additional water may need to be instilled between feedings.

Inserting a Nasogastric Tube

- Perform hand hygiene and observe other appropriate infection control procedures (e. g., clean gloves).
- Minimize discomfort by positioning the client appropriately, lubricating the tube with water-soluble lubricant, and working cooperatively with the client.
- Determine distance to insert tube: measure from the tip of the client's nose to the tip of the earlobe and then from the tip of the earlobe to the tip of the xiphoid.
- Have client hyperextend the neck until the tube passes into the nasopharynx. Never force the tube against resistance. Then, have the client flex the neck and swallow as the tube passes the glottis and into the esophagus.
- Confirm correct placement of the tube according to agency policy. Aspirate stomach contents, and check the pH, which should be acidic. Testing for bilirubin (absent if in the airway), X-ray examination, and

carbon dioxide detection (present if in the airway) may also be used. If a small-bore tube is used, leave the stylet or guidewire in place until correct position is verified by x-ray. If the stylet has been removed, never reinsert it while the tube is in place.

- Secure the tube appropriately to the client's nose or nose and cheek.

Removing a Nasogastric Tube

- If present, turn off the suction, and disconnect the tube from suction.
- Clamp the tubing.
- Remove the adhesive tape securing the tube to the nose.
- Apply clean gloves.
- Ask the client to take a deep breath and to hold it. Quickly and smoothly, withdraw the tube.

Administering a Tube Feeding

Before Administering the Feeding

- Assess the client for feelings of abdominal distention, belching, loose stools, flatus, or pain; assess the client for bowel sounds and allergies to foods in the feeding.
- Check the expiration date of the feeding.
- Position the client in Fowler's or right lateral position.
- Confirm correct placement of the tube.
  1. Aspirate 20 to 30 mL of gastrointestinal secretions. Gastric secretions tend to be a grassy-green, off-white, or tan color; intestinal fluid is stained with bile and has a golden yellow or brownish-green color.
  2. Measure the pH of aspirated fluid.
     - Gastric aspirates have a pH of 1 to 4 but may be as high as 6 if the client is receiving medications that control gastric acid.
     - Small intestine aspirates generally have a pH of 6 or higher.

    - Respiratory secretions have a pH of 7 or higher. There is a possibility of respiratory placement when the pH reading is as low as 6.
    - Therefore, when pH readings are 6 or higher, radiographic confirmation of tube location needs to be considered, especially in clients with diminished cough and gag reflexes.
- Aspirate all residual stomach contents; measure the amount. Check agency policy to determine whether to reinstill the contents or to continue the feeding.
- Deliver the feeding over the desired length of time.

During the Feeding

- If the client is on a continuous feeding, check the gastric residual every 4 to 6 hours or according to agency protocol.

After the Feeding

- Flush the tube with water.
- Clamp the tube before all of the rinse solution has run through.
- Have the client remain in Fowler's position or a slightly elevated right lateral position for at least 30 minutes.

Administering a Gastrostomy or Jejunostomy Feeding

Before the Feeding

- Position the client appropriately.
- Assess the peristomal skin.
- Lubricate tubes before inserting them into stomas.
- Aspirate, measure, test pH, and reinstill (if indicated) stomach or jejunal contents. Check agency policy to confirm whether the feeding is to be withheld if more than a specified amount of contents is aspirated.

Administer the Feeding

- Insert the barrel of a catheter-tip syringe in the end of the tube and hold it 7 to 15 cm (3 to 6 in.) above the ostomy opening.

- Slowly pour the feeding into the syringe and allow it to flow through the tube by gravity.
- Just before the syringe is empty, add 30 mL of water.
- If the tube is to remain in place, hold it upright, remove the syringe, and then clamp or plug the tube to prevent leakage.
- If a catheter was inserted for the feeding, remove it.

After the Feeding

- Have the client remain in Fowler's position or a slightly elevated right lateral position for at least 30 minutes.
- Clean the peristomal skin, and inspect for irritation.
- Apply peristomal skin protectants and appropriate dressings.

Special Care for Older Adults

- Physiologic changes associated with aging may make the older adult more vulnerable to complications associated with enteral feedings. Decreased gastric emptying may necessitate checking frequently for gastric residual. Diarrhea from administering the feeding too fast or too high concentration of the feeding may cause dehydration in the older adult. If the feeding has a high concentration of glucose, assess for hyperglycemia, because with aging there is decreased ability to handle increased glucose levels.
- Conditions such as hiatal hernia and diabetes mellitus may cause the stomach to empty more slowly. This increases the risk of aspiration in a client receiving a tube feeding. Checking for gastric residual more frequently can help document this if it is an ongoing problem. Changing the formula, altering the rate of administration, repositioning the client, or obtaining a primary care provider's order for a medication to increase stomach emptying may resolve this problem.

5. Urinary Elimination

Assess to Determine

- Client's usual patterns and frequency of urination. Ask at what approximate times voiding occurs each day.

Note Recent Alterations in Voiding

- Passage of unusually large or small amounts of urine
- Voiding at more frequent intervals
- Trouble getting to the bathroom in time or feeling of urgency to void
- Painful voiding
- Difficulty starting urine stream
- Frequent dribbling of urine or feeling of bladder fullness associated with voiding small amounts of urine
- Reduced force of stream
- Accidental leakage of urine; if so, when this occurs (e.g., when coughing, laughing, or sneezing; at night; during the day)

Obtain the Medical History of Urinary Elimination Problems

- Urinary tract infections of the kidney, bladder, or urethra
- Urinary calculi
- Urinary tract surgery, such as kidney surgery, bladder surgery, prostate removal, or other surgical procedures that alter urinary routes (e.g., ureterostomy)
- Cardiovascular disease, such as hypertension or heart disease
- Chronic diseases that alter urinary characteristics or impair urinary function, such as diabetes mellitus, neurologic disease (e.g., multiple sclerosis), and cancer

Assess the Volume and Characteristics of the Client's Urine

- Time when the client last voided and the amount (Volumes of less than 30 mL or more than 500 mL per hour must be reported immediately.)

- Dark, cloudy, or discolored urine
- Presence of mucous plugs
- Offensive odor

Determine Factors Influencing Urinary Elimination

- *Medications.* Any medications that could increase urinary output (e.g., diuretics) or cause retention of urine (e.g., anticholinergic-antispasmodic drugs, antidepressant-antipsychotic drugs, antiparkinsonism drugs, antihistamines, antihypertensives) or that may discolor urine (e.g., multivitamins, phenytoin, phenothiazines). Note specific medication and dosage.
- *Fluid intake.* Amount and kind of fluid taken each day (e.g., six glasses of water, three cups of coffee, two cola drinks with or without caffeine).
- *Environmental factors.* Any problems with toileting (mobility, dexterity with clothing, toilet seat too low, facility without grab bar).
- *Presence of long-term catheter.* How the client cares for the catheter, any discomfort with it or other problems, and how the nurse can help manage it.
- *Diagnostic procedures.* Recent procedures, such as cystoscopy or spinal anesthetic.

Determine the Presence of Pain

- *Bladder pain.* Pain over the suprapubic region
- *Kidney or flank pain.* Pain between ribs and ilium, which may spread to the abdomen and be associated with nausea and vomiting, or pain at the costovertebral angle, which may radiate to the umbilicus
- *Ureteral pain.* Pain in the back, which may radiate to abdomen, upper thigh, testes, or labia

Review Data from Diagnostic Tests and Examinations

- pH under 4.5 or over 8
- Specific gravity under 1.010 or over 1.025
- Presence of glucose or acetone
- Presence of occult or visible blood

- Presence of protein, urobilinogen, or nitrite
- Presence of microorganisms
- Presence of obstructions
- Blood serum: blood urea nitrogen, creatinine, sodium, potassium

Urinary Catheterization

- Use strict aseptic technique.
- For a retention catheter, test the balloon before insertion to see that it is intact. However, pretesting silicone catheters is *not* recommended.
- Lubricate the insertion tip of the catheter.
- Obtain assistance for a client who needs help to maintain the required position.
- For females: Clean the perineal area, keeping the labia apart once the meatus is cleaned.
- For males: Retract the foreskin of an uncircumcised client, and keep it back during the catheterization. Lift the penis perpendicular to the body before catheterization.
- Pick up and insert the catheter with your uncontaminated, sterile, gloved hand.
- Do not force a catheter beyond a major resistance.
- Before inflating the balloon of the retention catheter, insert the catheter an additional 2.5 to 5 cm (1 to 2 in.) beyond the point at which urine began to flow.
- Inflate the balloon with no more fluid than the balloon size indicates.
- After balloon inflation, apply slight tension on the catheter to check that the balloon is well anchored in the bladder; then move the catheter slightly back into the bladder.
- Secure the catheter to the client appropriately.
- Assess the amount, color, and clarity of the urine.
- Make sure the drainage system allows free flow of urine and is well sealed or closed.

Removing a Retention Catheter

- Wear gloves.
- Deflate the balloon completely before removing it from the urethra.
- Observe the intactness of the catheter.
- Measure the urine in the drainage bag.
- Assess the frequency and amount of urine voided after catheter removal.

Special Care for Older Adults

The following conditions are etiologic factors in problems with urinary elimination in elders:

- Many older men have enlarged prostate glands, which can cause retention and incontinence of urine.
- Women past menopause have decreased estrogen, which results in a decrease in perineal tone and support of bladder, vagina, and supporting tissues. This often results in urgency and stress incontinence and can even increase the incidence of urinary tract infections.
- Increased stiffness and pain in joints, previous joint surgery, and neuromuscular problems can impair mobility and often make it difficult to get to the bathroom.
- Cognitive impairment, such as in dementia, often prevents the person from understanding the need to urinate and the actions needed to perform the activity. The following interventions may improve these conditions:
  - Medications or surgery to relieve obstructions in men and strengthen support in the urogenital area in women
  - Behavioral training for better bladder control
  - Providing safe, easy access to the bathroom or bedside commode, whether at home or in an institution; making sure the room is well lit, environment is safe, and the proper assistive devices are within reach (such as walkers, canes)

- Habit training, such as taking the person to the bathroom at a regular, scheduled time can often work very well with cognitively impaired persons

- When catheterizing an older adult, be very attentive to problems of limited movement, especially in the hips. Arthritis or previous hip or knee surgery may limit the client's movement and cause discomfort. Modify the position as needed to perform the procedure safely and comfortably. For women, obtain the assistance of another nurse to flex and hold client's knees and hips as necessary or place her in a modified Sims' position.

6. Fecal Elimination

Assess to Determine

- *Defecation pattern.* What are the frequency and time of day of the client's defecation? Has this pattern changed recently? Does it ever change? If so, does the client know what factors affect it?

- *Behavioral patterns.* The client's use of laxatives, fluids, and exercise to maintain the normal defecation pattern? What routines does the client follow to maintain the usual defecation pattern (e.g., prune juice with breakfast)?

- *Diet.* What foods does the client believe affect defecation? What foods does the client typically eat? What food does the client always avoid? Does the client take meals at regular times?

- *Fluid intake.* What amount and kind of fluid does the client take each day (e.g., four glasses of water, two cups of coffee)?

- *Exercise.* What is the client's usual daily exercise pattern? Obtain specific details; avoid asking whether the client's exercise is sufficient because people's ideas of what is sufficient differ.

- *Use of elimination aids.* What routines does the client follow to maintain usual defecation pattern? Does the client use natural aids (e.g., specific foods or fluids), laxatives, or enemas to maintain elimination?

- *Medications.* Has the client taken any medications that could affect the gastrointestinal tract (e.g., iron supplements, antihistamines in cold preparations, antacids, narcotic analgesics)?
- *Pertinent illness or surgery.* Has the client had any surgery or illness that affects the intestinal tract? Are any ostomies (e.g., colostomy or ileostomy) present?

Assess the Client's

- *Vital signs* (pulse, respirations, and blood pressure) for baseline data, particularly before administering enemas or digitally removing a fecal impaction.
- *Abdominal distention.* Distention appears as an overall outward protuberance of the abdomen, with the skin appearing tight and tense. When palpated, the abdomen feels firm. Measure a distended abdomen at the level of the umbilicus by placing a tape measure around the body. Repeated measurements indicate whether the distention is increasing or decreasing.
- *Bowel sounds.* Auscultate all four abdominal quadrants for 5 to 15 seconds to determine the degree of activity or frequency of sounds.
- *Consistency and color of feces.* Normal feces are brown and formed but soft and moist. Note color of feces. For example, black, tarry feces may indicate the presence of blood from the stomach or small intestine; acholic (pale) feces usually indicate the absence of bile; and green or orange stools may indicate the presence of an intestinal infection. Food may also affect the color of feces; for example, beets can color stool red or sometimes green. Medications, too, can alter the color of feces; iron, for example, can make stool black.
- *Presence of constipation, diarrhea, or fecal incontinence.*
- *Perianal region and anus.* Inspect these areas for discoloration, inflammations, scars, lesions, fissures, fistulas, or hemorrhoids. Note the color, size, location, and consistency of any lesion.

- *Presence of abdominal or rectal pain.*
- *Presence of flatulence and signs associated with flatulence,* such as eructations (burping) and their frequency and the passage of flatus by the rectum. Also assess respiratory rate. Flatulence can cause pressure on the diaphragm, resulting in difficult respirations.

Identify Clients at Risk for Developing Fecal Elimination Problems

- Clients who have insufficient fluid or roughage in the diet
- Clients who do not exercise sufficiently
- Clients who use constipating medications
- Clients who ingest excessive gas-forming foods

Administering an Enema

For All Enemas

- Determine the type and purpose of the enema and whether a primary care provider's order is required.
- Position the client appropriately.
- Wear clean gloves.
- Assess the returns.

Cleansing Enema

- Use the correct type, amount, and temperature of solution.
- To remove air, flush the tubing before administering the enema.
- Lubricate the rectal tube before insertion.
- Direct the insertion tube toward the client's umbilicus.
- Ask the client to take a deep breath during tube insertion.
- Hold the solution container at the correct height.
- Administer the solution slowly, and start and stop the flow of solution temporarily if the client complains of cramping.

Retention Enema

- Instruct client to try to retain the enema at least 30 minutes.

Special Care for Older Adults

- Older adults may fatigue easily.
- Older adults may be more susceptible to fluid and electrolyte imbalances. Use tap water enemas with great caution.
- Monitor the client's tolerance during the procedure, watching for vagal episodes and dysrhythmias.
- Protect the older adult's skin from prolonged exposure to moisture.
- Assist the older adult with perineal care as indicated.

7. Pressure Areas

Assess to Determine

- The client's need for supportive devices, such as pillows, rolled or folded towels, foam supports, footboard, hand rolls, wrist splints, or sandbags by assessing the following in the client:
  - *Adipose tissue.* A client who has ample adipose tissue generally requires less support and cushioning than the emaciated person does while in a back-lying position, but greater support to maintain a lateral position.
  - *Skeletal structure.* Both the amount and the type of support needed vary according to the individual's skeletal structure. A person with a marked lumbar lordosis requires more lumbar support than one with a slight lumbar curvature.
  - *Health status.* A person who has flaccid or spastic paralysis requires supportive devices.
  - *Discomfort.* A person who experiences pain during movement requires more support during movement than one who can move without pain. A person who

is unconscious is unable to indicate discomfort and needs appropriate support and change of position at least every 2 hours.

- *Skin condition.* People who have nutritional problems or impaired circulation require more cushioning of the pressure points to prevent skin breakdown than do healthy people.
- *Ability to move.* People who can move in bed can change position frequently. The client who is unable to move (e.g., the unconscious client) requires support and positioning.
- *Hydration.* Dehydrated clients are at greater risk of pressure ulcer formation than well-hydrated clients and therefore need more support under pressure areas.

Assess the Client's

- Strength and ability to move before the change of position, and obtain assistance as required. Appropriate assistance reduces the risk of muscle strain and body injury to both the client and nurse.
- Pressure areas of the body for any pale or reddened spots. This discoloration, which can be caused by impaired blood circulation to the area, should disappear in a few minutes when pressure relief restores circulation. See Figure 3–1 for the location of pressure areas.
- Pressure areas of the body for abrasions and excoriations. An abrasion (wearing away of the skin) can occur when skin rubs against a sheet, such as when the client is pulled. Excoriations (loss of superficial layers of the skin) can occur when the skin has prolonged contact with body secretions or excretions, or with dampness in skinfolds.
- Classify pressure ulcers if present. Pressure ulcers are described as follows (European Pressure Ulcer Advisory Panel and National Pressure Ulcer Advisory Panel, 2009). *Category* is the most current term used to

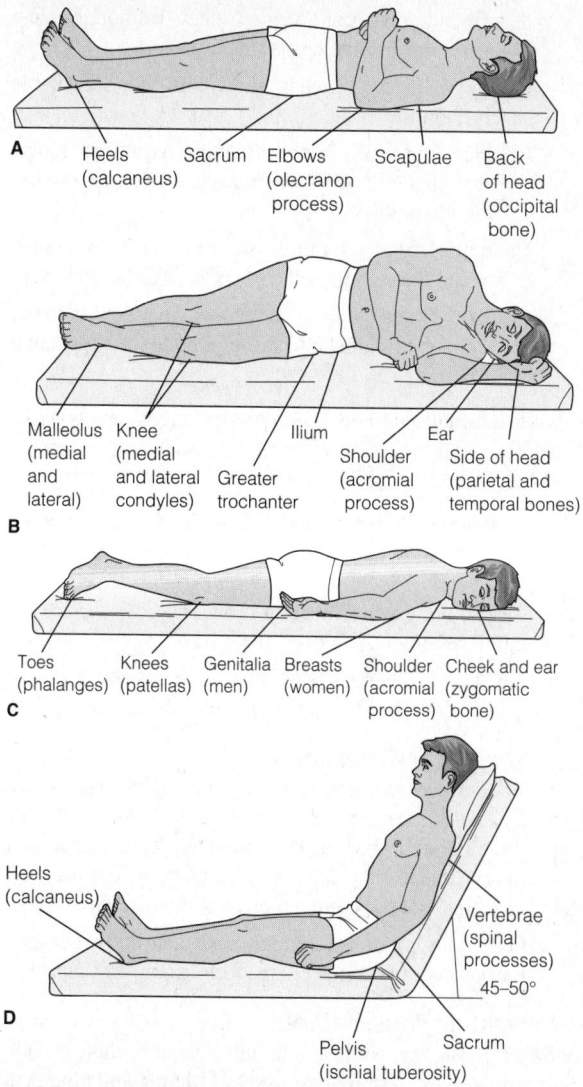

Figure 3–1 ■ Body pressure areas in **A**, supine position; **B**, lateral position; **C**, prone position; **D**, Fowler's position.

describe the different levels of ulcers (although many organizations use the terms *stage* or *grade*):

Category/Stage I: Intact skin with nonblanchable erythema

Category/Stage II: Partial-thickness skin loss (abrasion, blister, or shallow crater) involving the epidermis and possibly the dermis

Category/Stage III: Full-thickness skin loss may extend through the subcutaneous layer to the fascia

Category/Stage IV: Full-thickness skin loss with tissue necrosis or damage to muscle, bone, or supporting structures

Both international and U.S. pressure ulcer panels agree to these four categories/stages of pressure ulcers. In the U.S., two additional levels are used.

- Unstageable/Unclassified: Full thickness skin or tissue loss - depth unknown. The actual depth of the ulcer is completely obscured by slough (yellow or white tissue) and/or eschar (black or brown necrotic tissue) but it will be either a category/stage III or IV.
- Suspected Deep Tissue Injury - depth unknown. Purple area of discolored intact skin or blood-filled blister.

Palpate (with Warm Hands)

- The surface temperature of the skin over pressure areas. Normally, the temperature is the same as that of the surrounding skin. Increased temperature is abnormal and may be due to inflammation or blood trapped in the area. A decreased temperature indicates impaired circulation.
- Over bony prominences and dependent body areas for the presence of edema. Edema feels spongy on palpation.

Preventing Pressure Ulcers

Several risk assessment tools are available that provide the nurse with systematic means of identifying clients at high risk for pressure ulcer development.

The tool chosen for use should include data collection in the areas of immobility, incontinence, nutrition, and level of consciousness. One example, the Braden Scale, is shown in Figure 3–2.

Treating Pressure Ulcers

- Minimize direct pressure on the ulcer. Reposition the client at least every 2 hours. Make a schedule, and record position changes on the client's chart.
- Reduce friction on intact skin by using proper lifting and moving techniques.
- Reduce shearing force by keeping the head of the bed flat or elevated to a maximum of 30 degrees, unless contraindicated by the client's condition.
- Teach the client to move, even if only slightly, to relieve pressure.
- Encourage ambulation or sitting in a wheelchair as the client's condition permits.
- Provide range-of-motion exercises as the client's condition permits.
- Clean the pressure ulcer daily. Use a method consistent with the stage of the ulcer and agency protocol.
- Dress the ulcer. Refrain from using antiseptics, such as alcohol, that are vasoconstrictors and reduce blood flow to the area.

Special Care for Older Adults

- If the client cannot keep weight off the pressure ulcer, use pressure-relieving devices, such as foam gel pads or mattresses or specialty beds.
- Hold wrinkled skin taut during application of a transparent dressing. Obtain assistance if needed.
- Skin is more fragile and can easily tear with removal of tape (especially adhesive tape). Use paper tape and tape remover as indicated, keeping tape use to the

BRADEN SCALE FOR PREDICTING PRESSURE SORE RISK

Patient's Name _____ Evaluator's Name _____

					Date of Assessment			
SENSORY PERCEPTION Ability to respond meaningfully to pressure-related discomfort	**1. Completely Limited:** Unresponsive (does not moan, flinch, or grasp) to painful stimuli, due to diminished level of consciousness or sedation, OR limited ability to feel pain over most of body surface.	**2. Very Limited:** Responds only to painful stimuli. Cannot communicate discomfort except by moaning or restlessness, OR has a sensory impairment which limits the ability to feel pain or discomfort over 1/2 of body.	**3. Slightly Limited:** Responds to verbal commands but cannot always communicate discomfort or need to be turned, OR has some sensory impairment which limits ability to feel pain or discomfort in 1 or 2 extremities.	**4. No Impairment:** Responds to verbal commands. Has no sensory deficit which would limit ability to feel or voice pain or discomfort.				
MOISTURE Degree to which skin is exposed to moisture	**1. Constantly Moist:** Skin is kept moist almost constantly by perspiration, urine, etc. Dampness is detected every time patient is moved or turned.	**2. Moist:** Skin is often but not always moist. Linen must be changed at least once a shift.	**3. Occasionally Moist:** Skin is occasionally moist, requiring an extra linen change approximately once a day.	**4. Rarely Moist:** Skin is usually dry; linen requires changing only at routine intervals.				
ACTIVITY Degree of physical activity	**1. Bedfast:** Confined to bed.	**2. Chairfast:** Ability to walk severely limited or nonexistent. Cannot bear own weight and/or must be assisted into chair or wheelchair.	**3. Walks Occasionally:** Walks occasionally during day but for very short distances, with or without assistance. Spends majority of each shift in bed or chair.	**4. Walks Frequently:** Walks outside the room at least twice a day and inside room at least once every 2 hours during waking hours.				
MOBILITY Ability to change and control body position	**1. Completely Immobile:** Does not make even slight changes in body or extremity position without assistance.	**2. Very Limited:** Makes occasional slight changes in body or extremity position but unable to make frequent or significant changes independently.	**3. Slightly Limited:** Makes frequent though slight changes in body or extremity position independently.	**4. No Limitations:** Makes major and frequent changes in position without assistance.				

NUTRITION Usual food intake pattern	**1. Very Poor:** Never eats a complete meal. Rarely eats more than 1/3 of any food offered. Eats 2 servings or less of protein (meat or dairy products) per day. Takes fluids poorly. Does not take a liquid dietary supplement, OR is NPO and/or maintained on clear liquids or IV's for more than 5 days.	**2. Probably Inadequate:** Rarely eats a complete meal and generally eats only about 1/2 of any food offered. Protein intake includes only 3 servings of meat or dairy products per day. Occasionally will take a dietary supplement, OR receives less than optimum amount of liquid diet or tube feeding.	**3. Adequate:** Eats over half of most meals. Eats a total of 4 servings of protein (meat, dairy products) each day. Occasionally will refuse a meal, but will usually take a supplement if offered, OR is on a tube feeding or TPN regimen, which probably meets most of nutritional needs.	**4. Excellent:** Eats most of every meal. Never refuses a meal. Usually eats a total of 4 or more servings of meat and dairy products. Occasionally eats between meals. Does not require supplementation.				
FRICTION AND SHEAR	**1. Problem:** Requires moderate to maximum assistance in moving. Complete lifting without sliding against sheets is impossible. Frequently slides down in bed or chair, requiring frequent repositioning with maximum assistance. Spasticity, contractures, or agitation leads to almost constant friction.	**2. Potential Problem:** Moves feebly or requires minimum assistance. During a move skin probably slides to some extent against sheets, chair, restraints, or other devices. Maintains relatively good position in chair or bed most of the time but occasionally slides down.	**3. No Apparent Problem:** Moves in bed and in chair independently and has sufficient muscle strength to lift up completely during move. Maintains good position in bed or chair at all times.					
				Total Score				

Figure 3–2 ■ Braden scale for predictinig pressure sore risk.

Copyright © Barbara Breden and Nancy Bergstrom, 1988. Reprinted with permission.

minimum required. Use extreme caution during tape removal.

- Older adults in long-term care facilities often have immobility, malnutrition, and incontinence—all of which increase the risk for development of skin breakdown.
- Skin breakdown can occur as quickly as within 2 hours, so assessments should be done with each repositioning of the client.
- A thorough assessment of a client's heels should be done every shift. The skin can break down quickly from friction of movement in bed. (See Table 3–1 for pressure ulcer dressings.)

References

European Pressure Ulcer Advisory Panel and National Pressure Ulcer Advisory Panel. (2009). *Prevention and treatment of pressure ulcers: Quick reference guide*. Washington DC: National Pressure Ulcer Advisory Panel.

Table 3–1 Selected Types of Wound Dressings

Dressing	Description	Purpose	Indications
Transparent film	Adhesive plastic, semipermeable, nonabsorbent dressings allow exchange of oxygen between the atmosphere and wound bed. Impermeable to bacteria and water.	Protection against contamination and friction; maintain a clean, moist surface that facilitates cellular migration; provide insulation by preventing fluid evaporation; facilitate wound assessment	Intravenous dressing Central line dressing Superficial wounds Pressure ulcers category/stage I
Impregnated nonadherent	Woven or nonwoven cotton or synthetic materials impregnated with petrolatum, saline, zinc-saline, antimicrobials, or other agents. Require secondary dressings to secure them in place, retain moisture, and provide wound protection.	Cover, soothe, and protect partial- and full-thickness wounds without exudate	Postoperative dressing over staple/sutures Superficial burns
Hydrocolloids	Waterproof adhesive wafers, pastes, or powders. Inner adhesive layer has particles that absorb exudates and form a hydrated gel over the wound; outer film provides an occlusive seal.	Absorb exudate; produce a moist environment that facilitates healing but does not cause maceration of surrounding skin; protect the wound from bacterial contamination, foreign debris, and urine or feces; and prevent shearing	Pressure ulcers category/stage II–IV Autolytic debridement of eschar Partial thickness wounds

(continued)

Table 3–1 Selected Types of Wound Dressings *(continued)*

Dressing	Description	Purpose	Indications
Clear absorbent acrylic dressing	Transparent absorbent wafer. Acrylic layer absorbs exudates and evaporates the excess off the transparent membrane.	Maintains a transparent membrane for easy wound bed assessment, provides bacterial and shearing protection; maintains moist wound healing; can be used with alginates to provide packing to deeper wound beds	Pressure ulcers Skin tears Venous stasis ulcers Surgical wounds Wounds undergoing chemical debridement agents
Hydrogels	Glycerin- or water-based nonadhesive jellylike sheets, granules, or gels are oxygen-permeable, unless covered by a plastic film. Require secondary occlusive dressing.	Liquefy necrotic tissue or slough, rehydrate the wound bed, and fill in dead space	Pressure ulcers Skin tears Partial-thickness wounds
Collagen	Gels, pastes, powders, granules, sheets, sponges derived from animal sources, often cow or pig.	Assists with stopping bleeding, helps recruit cells into the wound and stimulates their proliferation to facilitate healing.	Clean, moist wounds

Polyurethane foams	Nonadherent hydrocolloid dressings. Require secondary dressings to obtain an occlusive environment. Surrounding skin must be protected to prevent maceration.	Absorb up to heavy amounts of exudate; provide and maintain moist wound healing	Light to highly exudating wounds Pressure ulcers Skin tears Venous stasis ulcers Surgical wounds Wounds undergoing chemical debridement agents
Alginates (exudate absorbers)	Nonadherent dressings of powder, beads or granules, ropes, sheets, or paste conform to the wound surface and absorb up to 20 times their weight in exudate. Require a secondary dressing.	Provide moist wound surface by interacting with exudate to form a gelatinous mass; absorb exudate; eliminate dead space or pack wounds; support debridement	Pressure ulcers Skin tears Venous stasis ulcers Surgical wounds Wounds undergoing chemical debridement agents

8. Healing Wounds

Assess to Determine

Appearance

- Inspect color of wound and surrounding area and approximation of wound edges.

Size

- Note size and location of dehiscence, if present. For wounds healing by secondary intention, measure the length, width, and depth in centimeters.

Drainage

- Observe location, color, consistency, odor, and degree of saturation of dressings. Note number of gauzes saturated or diameter of drainage on gauze.

Swelling

- Wearing gloves, palpate wound edges for tension and tautness of tissues; minimal to moderate swelling is normal in early stages of wound healing.

Pain

- Expect postoperative pain for 3 to 5 days; persistent severe pain or sudden onset of severe pain may indicate hemorrhaging or infection.

Drains or Tubes

- Inspect drain security and placement, amount and character of drainage, and functioning of collecting apparatus, if present.

Changing a Dry Sterile Dressing

- Support the adjacent skin when removing adhesive tape.
- Pull tape toward the wound rather than away from it.
- Wear clean gloves when removing moist outer dressings.
- Use sterile forceps or gloves to remove inner dressings.
- Support a drain appropriately when removing dressings.
- Use a separate swab for each cleaning stroke.
- Clean the wound from the cleanest to the least clean area.

- Clean a drain site after cleaning the incision.
- Dry the area around the wound appropriately.
- Assess the wound appearance and drainage accurately.
- Apply sufficient dressings to cover the wound and absorb drainage.
- Secure the dressing with tape or wrapping gauze, as appropriate.

Applying Damp-to-Damp Dressings

- Before the dressing change, medicate the client for pain as indicated.
- Maintain asepsis.
- Verify the ordered solution, and check agency policy about cleaning the wound.
- Assess the wound appearance and drainage.
- Thoroughly saturate the mesh gauze with solution, and then wring out excess moisture.
- Make sure all depressions and grooves of the wound are packed with the gauze.
- Cover the damp dressings appropriately. Do not apply an airtight occlusive covering.
- To keep the gauze damp, change or remoisten with saline.
- Although gauze is much less expensive than advanced dressings (e.g., polymers, alginates, collagens), the cost per week can be higher due to the number of dressing changes required.

Special Care for Older Adults

- Older adults may need extra support during dressing changes, especially if arthritis, contractures, or tremors are present.
- Avoid constricting the client's circulation with a tight bandage or binder. Observe skin and bony prominences frequently for signs of impaired circulation. The risk for skin breakdown increases with age.

9. Postoperative Period

Assess to Determine

- *Vital signs: pulse, respirations, and blood pressure.* Compare results with data from the post-anesthesia room (PAR) and preoperative baseline data. Many hospitals have postoperative routines for regular assessment of clients. In some agencies, assessments are made every 15 minutes until vital signs stabilize, every hour thereafter the same day, and every 4 hours for the next 2 days. Body temperature is usually assessed every 4 hours for the first few days. *It is vital that the assessments be made as frequently as the person's condition requires.* An elevated temperature, along with other signs, can indicate infection of the respiratory tract, urinary tract, or incision. A rapid, weak pulse and increased respiratory rate along with other signs can indicate infection, hemorrhage, or shock. A lowered blood pressure along with other signs can indicate hemorrhage, shock, or pulmonary embolism.
- *Skin color and temperature.* The color of the lips and nail beds is an indicator of tissue perfusion (passage of blood through the capillaries). Pale, cyanotic, cool, and moist skin may be a sign of circulatory problems.
- *Level of consciousness.* During the early postoperative period, most clients are conscious but drowsy.
- *Bleeding.* Inspect the dressings for bleeding, and inspect the bedclothes underneath the client for pooled blood. When dressings are changed, inspect the wound for signs of localized infection.
- *Intravenous infusion.* Observe the type of solution, the amount in the bottle, the drip rate, and the venipuncture site. Determine additional solutions ordered.
- *Patency of drainage tubes.* Note also the amount, color, consistency, and character of the drainage.
- *Fluid balance.* Measure the client's fluid intake and output for at least 2 days or until fluid balance is stable without an intravenous infusion.

- *Pain or discomfort and when the client last received an analgesic.* Note the location and type of pain, and determine the cause. Pain is usually greatest 12 to 36 hours after surgery, decreasing on the second or third day. Analgesics are usually administered every 3 or 4 hours the first day, and by the third day most clients require only oral analgesics. Signs of acute pain include pallor, perspiration, tension, and reluctance to perform deep-breathing and coughing exercises or to move or ambulate.
- *Any difficulties with voiding and/or bladder distention.*
- *Return of peristalsis.* Auscultate the client's abdomen to confirm the return of peristalsis. Note the passage of flatus and stool.
- *Tolerance of food and fluids ingested.*

Determine Clinical Signs of Postoperative Complications

- *Pneumonia:* Elevated temperature, cough, expectoration of blood-tinged or purulent sputum, dyspnea, chest pain.
- *Atelectasis:* Marked dyspnea, cyanosis, pleural pain, tachycardia, increased respiratory rate, fever, productive cough, auscultatory crackling sounds.
- *Pulmonary embolism:* Sudden chest pain, shortness of breath, cyanosis, shock (tachycardia, low blood pressure).
- *Thrombophlebitis:* Aching, cramping pain; affected area is swollen, red, and hot to touch; vein feels hard; discomfort in calf when foot is dorsiflexed or when client walks (Homans' sign).
- *Thrombus or embolus:* Same as for pulmonary embolism; if lodged in heart or brain, assess cardiac or neurologic signs.
- *Urinary retention:* Fluid intake larger than output, inability to void or frequent voiding of small amounts, bladder distention, suprapubic discomfort, restlessness, bladder palpable above the pubic symphysis.

- *Urinary infection:* Burning sensation when voiding, urgency, cloudy urine, lower abdominal pain.
- *Constipation:* Absence of stool elimination, abdominal distention, and discomfort.
- *Tympanites:* Obvious abdominal distention, abdominal discomfort (gas pains), absence of bowel sounds.
- *Wound infection:* Purulent exudate, redness, tenderness, elevated body temperature, wound odor.
- *Wound dehiscence:* Increased incision drainage; tissues underlying skin become visible along parts of the incision.
- *Wound evisceration:* Opening of incision and visible protrusion of organs.

Managing Gastrointestinal Suction

- Confirm the placement of the nasogastric tube before establishing suction.
- Place an air vent appropriately, and maintain its patency by injecting air.
- Test the functioning of the suction system before connecting it.
- Prevent kinks or blockages in the tubing.
- Keep all connections well sealed.
- Inspect the flow of gastric secretions into the drainage bottle.
- Clean the nares around the nasogastric tube at least every 3 hours.
- Provide mouth care.

Irrigations

- Obtain the physician's order if needed.
- Confirm the placement of the tube before irrigation.
- Reconnect the tube, and attach it to suction after irrigating.
- Assess the amount and character of the drainage, client comfort, and abdominal distention.

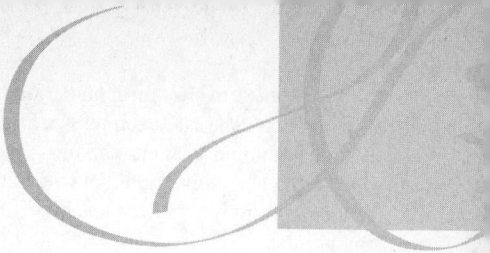

C. Teaching and Learning Guidelines

Teaching is a process designed to produce specific learning. The teaching and learning process involves dynamic interaction between the teacher and the learner. For teaching to be effective, trust must be established between the teacher and the learner, and communication must be open. Teaching is a five-step process similar to the nursing process:

1. Collect data; analyze client's learning strengths and deficits.
2. Make educational diagnoses.
3. Prepare teaching plan.
4. Implement teaching plan.
5. Evaluate client learning (effectiveness of teaching process).

Nurses teach in a variety of ways and settings. Teaching may be planned, as in preoperative teaching. Teaching may also result during an interaction with a client. For example, when caring for a postoperative client, you find the client tense and in pain. Although the client has patient-controlled analgesia, you assess that the client does not understand how to use the pump. As part of your professional responsibilities, you must first make the client comfortable by administering the appropriate pain medicine and then teach the client how to use the patient-controlled analgesia device.

Teaching can occur in many settings. In the hospital, teaching may be part of your daily client care. It may also be more formal, as in childbirth preparation classes or diabetes education classes. Teaching is a large part of home health and community health nursing. Teaching occurs in any location where nurses interact with clients.

When planning your client teaching, consider the following points:

- Learning requires energy and the ability to concentrate. Extreme anxiety or such physiologic factors as pain or sleep deprivation make it difficult for the client to learn. The nurse needs to consider the client's physical condition. The client who has been medicated for pain may or may not be ready for teaching. If the client is groggy from the medication, defer teaching; if, however, the pain medication has allowed the client to relax and become alert, this may be a good time to conduct a teaching session.
- Motivation is a powerful facilitator of learning. Clients who understand why they need to learn and who recognize the benefit of this knowledge are more likely to succeed. For example, the hazards of smoking are well known. Telling clients that quitting the habit will improve their health may not be sufficient; you must find out what is important to them so that the teaching is based on their learning needs, not yours.
- To maximize learning, create the best learning environment. It is often difficult to teach in a crowded hospital room. Roommates may have visitors or the television may be on, and privacy may not be possible. Attempt to modify the environment to promote learning. Plan to teach during quiet hours and when the client is comfortable and alert. Sometimes it is best to take the client to a quiet conference room.
- Establish rapport with the client before you begin instruction. Find out who the client is and what the client already knows. Build on the client's prior knowledge.
- Present your teaching in a form that the client can understand. Language and cultural differences may

affect learning. For the client who speaks a different language, arrange translator services. Be careful when using family or support system members as translators. If it is important for family members to be part of the learning process, avoid asking them to act as translators; they may be so busy translating that they cannot take in the information you present.

- Honor cultural differences. To establish rapport with the client and family, approach them with respect. Attempt to learn about the client's beliefs and values. Teaching that is in violation of cultural beliefs has little likelihood of succeeding. For more information on cultural issues, see Chapter 18 of *Fundamentals of Nursing*.
- Be certain to speak at the level the client can understand. Health care workers often speak in jargon. For example, a client may not understand what you mean when you say, "I'm going to straight cath you in order to get a sterile urine for C&S." You will need to explain this in terms with which the client is familiar and at the level that is appropriate for the client.
- Know your client. Choose your teaching strategy based on the client. Good teaching begins with client assessment. Determine what type of learner the client is, and orient your teaching according to this assessment. Is the client an auditory learner? If so, arrange a quiet time to talk. Is the client a visual learner? If so, discussion is not the best teaching strategy for this client. Instead, try drawings and pictures or videotapes. Is the client a hands-on learner, or is the material best presented in this fashion? Teaching a client how to self-administer an injection cannot be accomplished by merely talking about the technique. This type of teaching is best conducted by allowing the client to handle the syringe and medication.
- When teaching home care strategies, make sure you acquire adequate information about the home environment. Take the time to learn about the client so that the teaching is tailored to the client's situation. Suppose

you are the hospital nurse caring for a client who has fallen and broken her hip. She has had surgery, and you are preparing her for discharge home. If the client is using a walker, can she get into a narrow bathroom with her walker? If she cannot yet negotiate stairs, how will she manage at home if the bedroom and bath are upstairs and the kitchen downstairs? Interview the client so that your teaching can be geared to her situation. Maybe she needs a home health aide. You will not know if you do not ask, and if you do not ask, the client may be back in the hospital with further problems.

- Make sure you are teaching the right person. Suppose, for example, that a beginning nursing student is caring for a newly diagnosed client with diabetes and gives him detailed instruction on modifying his diet. However, when making a home visit, the nurse finds that none of this information is being used. The teaching had been directed to the wrong person because, as the client then informs the nurse, he does not do the shopping or the cooking. The nurse had failed to include the right person in her teaching. She should have asked the client's partner to participate in the diet instruction.
- Provide frequent feedback. Praise clients for what they have done well, and continue to work on areas that need improvement.

To summarize, effective teaching:

- Holds the learner's interest.
- Fosters a positive self-concept in the learner; learner believes learning is probable.
- Supports the learner with positive reinforcement.
- Makes partners of the learner and the teacher.
- Is accurate and current.
- Is appropriate for the learner's age, condition, and abilities.
- Is optimistic, positive, and nonthreatening.

Special Care for Older Adults

Teaching and Learning

Older adults often have chronic illnesses that require multiple treatments and/or medications. Health teaching focuses on the same areas as with other ages—health and wellness promotion and prevention of illness and accidents—but often the needs are greatest in learning to live with conditions that they have and to maintain optimal health and functioning. For elders to be motivated to learn, the material must be practical and have meaning for them individually, especially if the information is new to them. Special considerations in teaching older adults are as follows:

- Make health promotion a priority need and include the following areas:
  - Exercise
  - Nutrition
  - Safety habits
  - Regular health check-ups
  - Understanding of medications
- Set achievable goals; involve the client and family.
- If using visual aids, use large print and contrasting colors.
- Increase time for teaching, allow for rest periods.
- Repeat information if necessary.
- Use return demonstrations with psychomotor skills, such as teaching someone how to do insulin injections.
- Determine where older adults obtain most of their health information (newspapers, magazines, television).
- Use examples that they can relate to in their daily life.
- Be aware of sensory deficits, such as hearing and vision.
- Use the setting where the individual is most comfortable—either a group or one-on-one setting.

- If noncompliance is a problem, investigate the cause—it could be due to lack of finances, transportation problems, or poor access to medical care.

Older adults come with a lifetime of experiences and learned knowledge of their own. Respect this, and always have them use their strengths to work with any problems. Positive reinforcement and ongoing evaluation of what has been taught are important factors in effective health teaching with older adults.

D. MEDICATIONS

Proper management of client medications is essential to safe patient care. A survey on use of drugs and medications, any allergies, or reports of problems with medications should be part of every nursing history. Safety consciousness should be uppermost in your mind when you administer medications. Always practice the "rights" for accurate medication administration:

- Right client
- Right medication
- Right dose
- Right time
- Right route
- Right documentation
- Right client education
- Right assessment
- Right evaluation
- Right to refuse

Check each medication thoroughly, and check the accuracy of the medication administration record with the primary care provider's order. A medication order must be complete. It must contain the client's name, the date, the medication, dose, route, method of administration, and signature of the prescriber. If any section of the order is unclear, difficult to read, or missing, contact the primary care provider. See Chapter 35 of *Fundamentals of Nursing* for a thorough discussion of medications, and remember, client safety must come first!

Check the medication against the order to be certain you are using the right medication. Many medications have similar names. Often a medication may be ordered in a trade name but be available in a generic form. Consult a drug guide to check for equivalency. With newer medications, you may need to consult a pharmacist for this type of information. After you have completed your preparation of the medication, check again for accuracy before you administer the medication to the client. Identify the client before administering any medication. Check the client's name band against the medication administration record. If the name band is missing, ask the client to identify himself or herself, or ask another nurse to verify the client's identity. The Joint Commission requires a nurse to use at least two client identifiers whenever administering medications. Neither identifier can be the client's room number. Acceptable identifiers may be the person's name, assigned identification number, telephone number, photograph, or other person-specific identifier. Check agency policy.

Your responsibility does not end once you administer the medication. A record must be kept of all medications administered. Promptly chart them after you administer them. When you get busy, it is tempting to postpone your charting. However, you run the risk that your preceptor will repeat the administration. Likewise, never chart a medication before giving it. When you chart, you are stating that you have prepared the medication and that the client has taken it. Too many things can go wrong if you prechart—the client may refuse, the client may be away from the unit at the prescribed time, or the client may even expire. Always chart that you have given the medication only after you have given it.

- Nurses who administer medications are responsible for their own actions. Question any order that you consider incorrect.

- Be knowledgeable about the medications you administer.
- Federal laws govern the uses of narcotics and barbiturates. Keep these medications in a locked place.
- Use only medications that are in a clearly labeled container.
- Return liquid medications that are cloudy or have changed color to the pharmacy.
- Do not leave medication at the bedside, with certain exceptions (e.g., nitroglycerin). Check agency policy.
- If a client vomits after taking an oral medication, report this to the nurse in charge.
- Take special precautions when administering certain medications; for example, have another nurse check the dosages of anticoagulants, insulin, and certain intravenous preparations.
- Most hospitals require new orders from the surgeon for the client's postsurgery care.
- When a medication is omitted for any reason, record the fact together with the reason.
- When a medication error is made, report it immediately to the nurse in charge.

Table 3–2 includes common abbreviations used in medication orders.

Special Care for Older Adults

Medications

- The physiologic changes associated with aging influence medication administration and effectiveness. Examples include altered memory, less acute vision, decrease in renal function, less complete and slower absorption from the gastrointestinal tract, and decreased liver function. Many of these changes enhance the possibility of cumulative effects and toxicity.

Table 3–2 Common Abbreviations Used in Medication Orders

Abbreviation	Explanation	Example of Administration Time
ac	before meals	0700, 1100, and 1700 hrs
ad lib	freely, as desired	
bid	twice a day	0900 and 2100 hrs
c̄	with	
cap	capsule	
elix	elixir	
g (G)	gram	
gr	grain	
gtt	drop	
h	an hour	
IM	intramuscular	
IV	intravenous	
m	minim	
mg	milligram	
mL (ml)	milliliter	
OD	right eye	
OS	left eye	
OU	both eyes	
pc	after meals	0900, 1300, and 1900 hrs
po	by mouth	
prn	when needed	
q	every	
QAM	every morning	1000 hrs
Rx	take, prescription	
s̄	without	
ss (s̄s̄)	one-half	
sup (supp)	suppository	
susp	suspension	
tid	three times a day	1000, 1400, and 1800 hrs

- Older adults usually require smaller dosages of drugs, especially sedatives and other central nervous system depressants.
- Older adults are mature adults capable of reasoning. The nurse therefore needs to explain the reasons for and the effects of the client's medications.
- Older adults may have a decreased muscle mass or muscle atrophy. A shorter needle may be needed. Assessment of appropriate injection site is critical.

1. Methods of Calculating Dosages

Four common formulas are used to calculate drug dosages. Any of the formulas can be used. You are encouraged to choose the method that works best for you. It is important to use one method consistently to avoid confusion in calculations and, thus, promote client safety. When calculating drug dosages, there are times when the nurse may need to round numbers. Box 3–1 reviews general guidelines for rounding.

Basic Formula

The **basic formula** for calculating drug dosages is commonly used and easy to remember:

D = Desired dose (i.e., dose ordered by primary care provider)

H = Dose on hand (i.e., dose on label of bottle, vial, ampule)

V = Vehicle (i.e., form in which the drug comes, such as tablet or liquid)

$$\text{Formula} = \frac{D \times V}{H} = \text{amount to administer}$$

Example

Order: Erythromycin 500 mg

On Hand: 250 mg in 5 mL

D = 500 mg H = 250 mg V = 5 mL

Box 3–1 Guidelines for Rounding Numbers in Drug Calculations Generally

- Quantities *greater than 1* are rounded to the nearest *tenth.*
- Quantities *less than 1* are rounded to the nearest *hundredth* (Olsen et al., 2008, p. 9).

To round to the nearest tenth:

- Look at the number in the hundredths place. If this number is 5 or greater, add 1 to the tenths place number. For example, 1.67 = 1.7. If the number in the hundredths place is less than 5, leave the number in the tenths place as is. For example, 1.63 = 1.6.

To round to the nearest hundredth:

- Look at the number in the thousandths place. If this number is 5 or greater, add 1 to the hundredths place number. For example, 0.825 = 0.83. If the number in the thousandths place is less than 5, leave the number in the hundredths place as is. For example, 0.823 = 0.82.

ORAL MEDICATIONS

- A capsule cannot be divided.
- Tablets that are scored (a line marked on the tablet) may be divided. A tablet must be scored by the manufacturer to be divided properly.
- For tablets that are *not* scored and capsules, it may not be realistic to administer the exact amount as calculated. For example, if the calculation for *x* results in 1.9 tablets or capsules, the nurse gives 2 tablets or capsules because it is unrealistic to accurately administer 1.9 tablets or capsules.
- If the oral medication is a liquid, the nurse checks to see if it is possible to administer an accurate dosage. This often depends on the syringes used to draw up the medication. For example, a tuberculin (TB) syringe is a 1-mL syringe that includes markings for hundredths of a milliliter. These syringes are often used in pediatrics because they can measure medications given in very small amounts. The nurse needs to pay attention to the

markings on the syringe. Some syringes (e.g., 3-mL) have calibrations where each line indicates one tenth of a milliliter. In contrast, the calibration lines for larger syringes (e.g., 10-mL) indicate a 0.2-mL increment. The nurse must select the proper size syringe for the calculated volume of medication.

PARENTERAL MEDICATIONS

- Rounding depends on the amount (i.e., less than or more than 1) and the syringe used. As indicated above, a TB syringe can be used for very small amounts (e.g., to the hundredth of a mL) and larger syringes would be used for rounding to a tenth of a milliliter.

IV INFUSION

- By gravity:
  - Round to the nearest whole number. For example, if the flow rate calculation equals 37.5 drops/minute, the nurse adjusts the flow rate to 38 drops/minute.
- By IV pump:
  - If the IV pump uses only whole numbers, round to the nearest whole number.
  - Some IV pumps used in critical care units can be set to a tenth of a rate (e.g., 11.1 mL/h). Round to the nearest tenth decimal point.

ROUNDING DOWN

- Rounding down may be used in pediatrics or when administering high-alert medications to adults. This type of rounding is done to avoid the danger of an overdose.
- To round down to hundredths, drop all of the numbers after the hundredth place. For tenths, drop all of the numbers after the tenth place, and for whole numbers, all of the numbers after the decimal. For example, 6.6477 rounded down to the nearest
  - Hundredth = 6.64.
  - Tenth = 6.6.
  - Whole number = 6.

Ratio and Proportion Method

The **ratio and proportion method** is considered the oldest method used for calculating dosage problems. The equation is set up with the known quantities on the left side (i.e., H [dose on hand] and V [form in which the drug comes]). The right side of the equation consists of the desired dose (i.e., D) and the unknown amount to administer (i.e., x). The equation looks like this:

$$H : V :: D : x$$

Once the equation is set up, multiply the extremes (i.e., H and x) and the means (i.e., V and D). Then solve for x.

Example

Order: Keflex 750 mg

On Hand: Keflex 250 mg capsules

$$H = 250 \text{ mg} : V = 1 \text{ capsule} : : D = 750 \text{ mg} : x$$

$$250 : 1 :: 750 : x$$

Multiply the extremes (i.e., H and x) and the means (V and D):

$$250x = 750$$

$$x = 3 \text{ tablets}$$

Fractional Equation Method

The **fractional equation method** is similar to ratio and proportion, except it is written as a fraction:

$$\frac{H}{V} = \frac{D}{x}$$

The formula consists of cross multiplying and solving for x:

$$\frac{H}{V} = \frac{D}{x}$$

$$Hx = DV$$

$$x = \frac{DV}{H}$$

Example

Order: Lanoxin 0.25 mg

On Hand: Lanoxin 0.125 mg tablets

$$\frac{0.125 \text{ mg}}{1 \text{ tablet}} = \frac{0.25 \text{ mg}}{x \text{ tablets}}$$

Cross multiply:

$$0.125\,x = 0.25$$

Solve for x:

$$\frac{\cancel{0.125}x}{\cancel{0.125}} = \frac{0.25}{0.125}$$

$$x = 2 \text{ tablets}$$

Dimensional Analysis Method

The **dimensional analysis method** is often used in the physical sciences where a quantity in one unit of measurement is converted to an equivalent quantity in a different unit of measurement by canceling matching units of measurement. One advantage of dimensional analysis is that only one equation is needed. The three components (D, H, and V) are still needed to solve the problem. However, when the units of measurement differ for D and H, the dimensional analysis method includes the conversion factor in the equation. The formula is as follows:

where V = vehicle; H = on hand; D = desired;
C = conversion factor:

$$V = \frac{V \times C(H) \times D}{H \times C(D) \times 1}$$

(drug label) × (conversion) × (drug order)

If the D and H are of the same unit of measurement, the conversion factor is not included in the equation.

Example

Order: Valsartan 120 mg

On Hand: Valsartan 40 mg tablets

1. On the *left* side of the equation, put the drug form [V] (e.g., tablet, capsule, mL) of *x*. For example: *x* tablet = .
2. On the *right* side of the equation, put the information related to the drug label. This information is put in the equation as a fraction. The information that matches the *x* quantity must be put in the *numerator*. The information about the numerator is placed in the *denominator*. Continuing the above example:

$$x \text{ tablet} = \frac{1 \text{ tablet}}{40 \text{ mg}}$$

3. Place the information about the conversion factor on the right side of the equation. In this example, the units are the same and there is no need for a conversion factor in the equation.
4. Next, find the information that matches the information in the denominator of the fraction. That is, the desired dose. In this case, that is milligrams and the order is for 120 mg. Add this information to the right side of the equation.

$$x \text{ tablet} = \frac{1 \text{ tablet} \times 120 \text{ mg}}{40 \text{ mg} \times 1}$$

5. Cancel like abbreviations on the *right* side of the equation. After doing this, the remaining measurement should match the one on the left side of the equation:

$$x \text{ tablet} = \frac{1 \text{ tablet} \times 120 \cancel{\text{mg}}}{40 \cancel{\text{mg}} \times 1}$$

Solve for x:

$$x = \frac{120}{40}$$

$$x = 3 \text{ tablets}$$

Example Using a Conversion Factor

Order: Dofetilide 0.5 mg

On Hand: 125 mcg capsules

$$x \text{ capsules} = \frac{1 \text{ capsule} \times 1{,}000 \text{ mcg} \times 0.5 \text{ mg}}{125 \text{ mcg} \times 1 \text{ mg} \times 1}$$

$$x \text{ capsules} = \frac{1 \text{ capsule} \times 1{,}000 \cancel{\text{mcg}} \times 0.5 \cancel{\text{mg}}}{125 \cancel{\text{mcg}} \times 1 \cancel{\text{mg}} \times 1}$$

$$x = \frac{500}{125}$$

$$x = 4 \text{ capsules}$$

2. Injection Techniques

Review Figures 3–1 to 3–4 for injection sites, types of injections, and injection techniques.

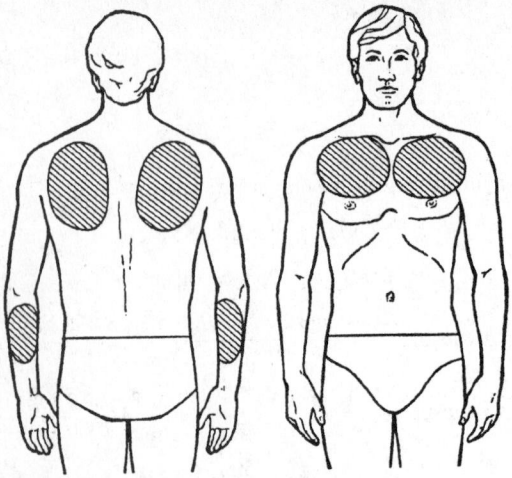

A

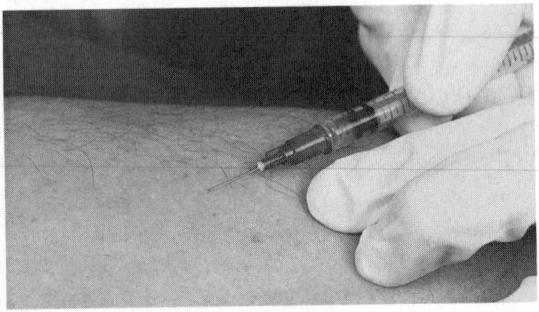

B

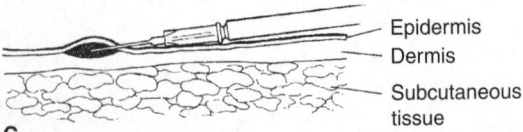

C

Figure 3–1 ■ **A,** Body sites commonly used for intradermal injections. For an intradermal injection: **B,** the needle enters the skin at a 15-degree angle; and **C,** the medication forms a bleb under the epidermis.

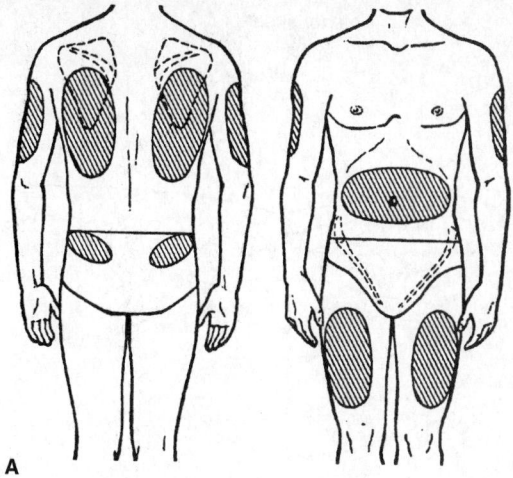

A

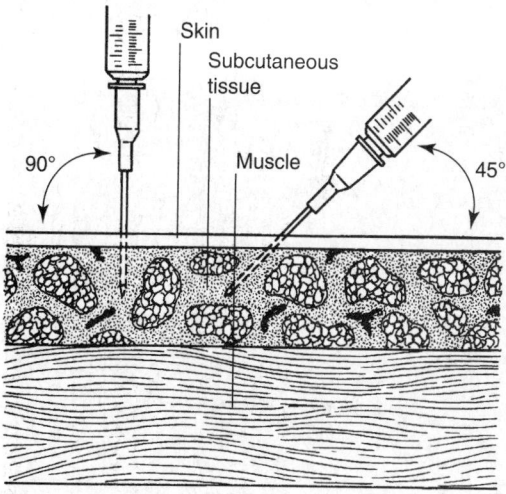

B

Figure 3–2 ■ **A,** Body sites commonly used for subcutaneous injections. **B,** Inserting a needle into the subcutaneous tissue using 90-degree and 45-degree angles.

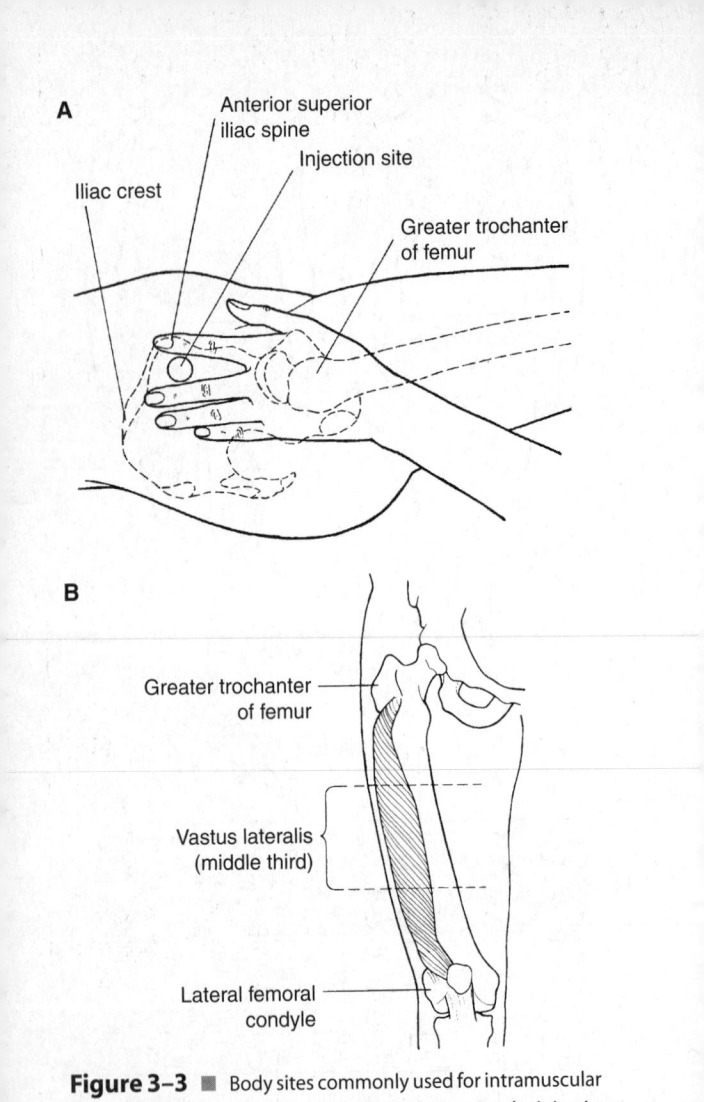

Figure 3–3 ■ Body sites commonly used for intramuscular injections. **A,** the ventrogluteal site for an intramuscular injection; **B,** the vastus lateralis site for an intramuscular injection. *(Continued)*

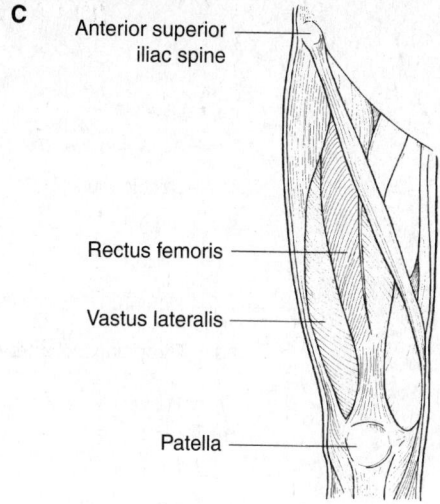

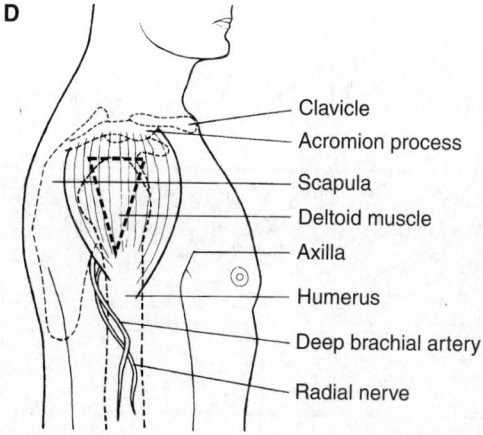

Figure 3–3 ■ Body sites commonly used for intramuscular injections. **C,** the rectus femoris muscle of the upper right thigh, used for intramuscular injections; **D,** the deltoid muscle of the upper arm, used for intramuscular injections. *(Continued)*

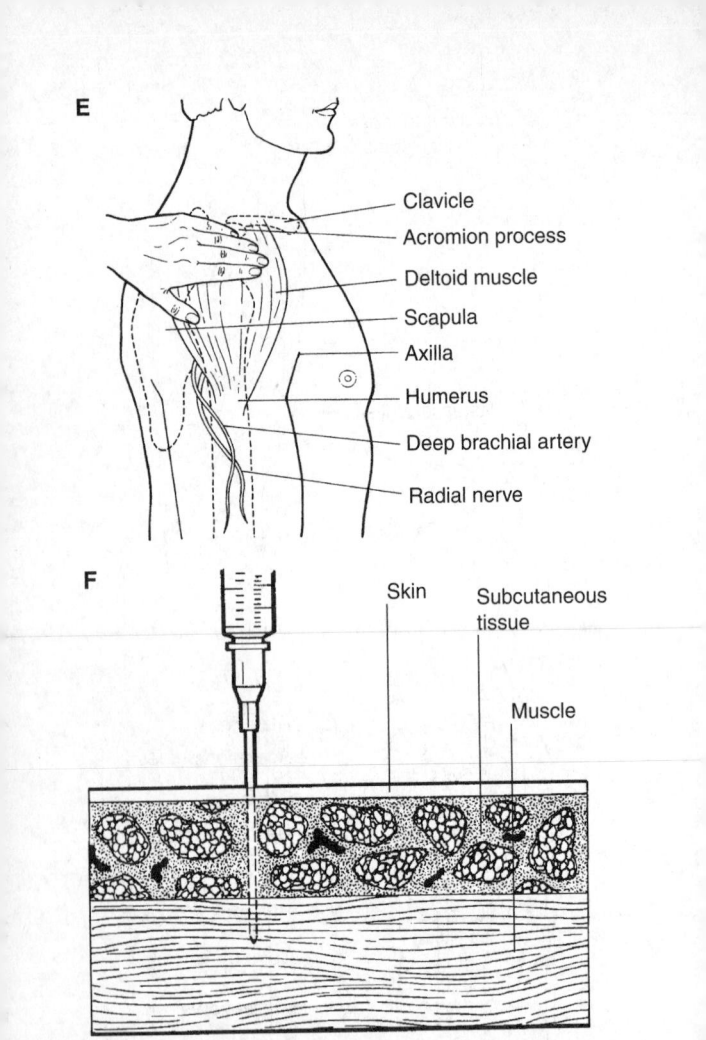

Figure 3–3 ■ Body sites commonly used for intramuscular injections. **E,** a method of establishing the deltoid muscle for an intramuscular injection; **F,** an intramuscular needle inserted into the muscle layer.

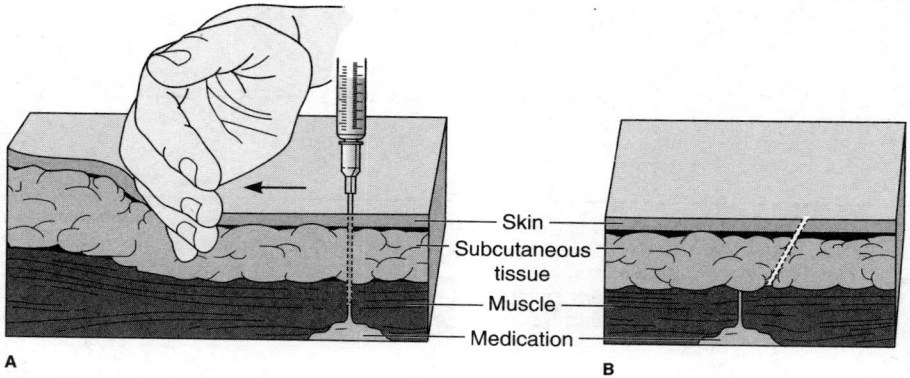

Figure 3–4 ■ Inserting an intramuscular needle at a 90-degree angle using the Z-track method: **A,** skin pulled to the side; **B,** skin released. ***Note:*** When the skin returns to its normal position after the needle is withdrawn, a seal is formed over the intramuscular site. This prevents seepage of the medication into the subcutaneous tissues and subsequent discomfort.

Table 3–3 Parenteral Medications

Route	Site	Needle Gauge	Needle Length	Syringe	Usual Amount	Angle used
Intradermal	Inner lower arm	# 25–27	¼ – 5/8″	1 mL TB syringe	0.1 mL	Parallel to skin surface
Subcutaneous	Outer aspect of upper arm	# 25	5/8″	2–3 mL syringe	0.5–1 mL	45 degrees
			3/8″			90 degrees
	Abdomen:					
	• Insulin	# 30	5/16″	0.3, 0.5, and 1 mL syringe	dependent on order or sliding scale	90 degrees
	• Heparin	# 25–26	3/8″	Lovenox-prefilled	0.5–1 mL	90 degrees
Intramuscular	Deltoid	# 23–25	1″	3–5 mL syringe	0.5–1 mL	90 degrees
	Ventrogluteal	# 21–22	1 ½″	3–5 mL syringe	1–3 mL	90 degrees

UNIT 4

DOCUMENTATION AND EVALUATION

A. Documentation
   1. Ethical and Legal Considerations
   2. Ensuring Confidentiality of Computer Records
   3. Charting Guidelines
   4. Essential Client Information
B. Documentation Formats
   1. Narrative
   2. SOAP
   3. Focus Charting (DAR)
C. Evaluation

A. Documentation

1. Ethical and Legal Considerations

The American Nurses Association Code of Ethics (2008) states that "... the nurse has a duty to maintain confidentiality of all patient information" (p. 152). The client's record is also protected legally as a private record of the client's care. Access to the record is restricted to health professionals involved in giving care to the client. The new HIPAA regulations maintain the privacy and confidentiality of protected health information (PHI). The student or graduate is bound by a strict ethical code and legal responsibility to hold all information in confidence.

2. Ensuring Confidentiality of Computer Records

Because of the increased use of electronic medical records (EMRs), health care agencies have developed policies and procedures to ensure the privacy and confidentiality of client information stored in computers. The following are some suggestions for ensuring the confidentiality and security of computerized records:

- A personal password is required to enter and sign off computer files.
- Do not share this password with anyone, including other health team members.
- After logging on, never leave a computer terminal unattended.

- Do not leave client information displayed on the monitor where others may see it.
- Shred all unneeded computer-generated worksheets.
- Know the facility's policy and procedure for correcting an entry error.
- Follow agency procedures for documenting sensitive material, such as a diagnosis of AIDS.

3. Charting Guidelines

DO

- Chart a change in a client's condition *and* show that follow-up actions were taken.
- Read the nurses' notes prior to care to determine if there has been a change in the client's condition.
- Be timely. A late entry is better than no entry; however, the longer the period of time between actual care and charting, the greater the suspicion.
- Use objective, specific, and factual descriptions.
- Correct charting errors.
- Chart all teaching.
- Record the client's actual words by putting quotes around the words.
- Chart the client's response to interventions.
- Review your notes—are they clear and do they reflect what you want to say?

DON'T

- Leave a blank space for a colleague to chart later.
- Chart in advance of the event (e.g., procedure, medication).
- Use vague terms (e.g., "appears to be comfortable," "had a good night").
- Chart for someone else.
- Record "patient" or "client" because it is their chart.

- Alter a record even if requested by a superior or a primary care provider.
- Record assumptions or words reflecting bias (e.g., "complainer," "disagreeable").

4. Essential Client Information

The following may assist you in selecting essential client information to record. Note that you should emphasize data that denote a change in the client's health status or behavior and data that indicate a deviation from what is usually expected.

1. Any behavior changes, for example,
   - Indications of strong emotions, such as anxiety or fear
   - Marked changes in mood
   - A change in level of consciousness, such as stupor
   - Regression in relationships with family or friends
2. Any changes in physical function, such as
   - Loss of balance
   - Loss of strength
   - Difficulty hearing or seeing
3. Any physical sign or symptom that
   - Is severe, such as severe pain
   - Tends to recur or persist
   - Deviates from normal, such as elevated body temperature
   - Gets worse, such as weight loss
   - Indicates faulty health habits, such as lice on the scalp
   - Is a known danger signal, such as a lump in the breast
4. Any nursing interventions provided, such as
   - Medications administered
   - Therapies

- Activities of daily living, if agency policy dictates
- Teaching clients self-care

5. Select data gathered from visits by a primary care provider or other members of the health team.

Reference

ANA. (2008). *Guide to the code of ethics for nurses.* Silver Spring, MD: Author.

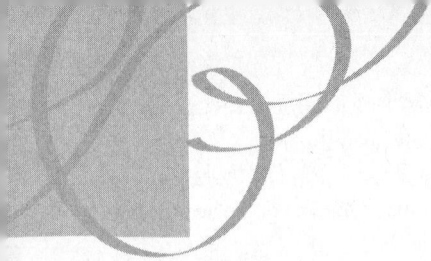

B. Documentation Formats

1. Narrative

Narrative charting consists of written notes that include routine care, normal findings, and client problems. There is no right or wrong order to the information, although chronological order is frequently used. Few institutions use only narrative charting today. When using narrative charting, it is important to organize the information in a clear, coherent manner. Using the nursing process as a framework is one way to do this. See following example:

Example of Organizing Narrative Charting

Situation: Client is postop day 2 after abdominal surgery.
Questions to ask yourself:

- What assessment data are relevant?
- What nursing interventions have I completed?
- What is my evaluation of the result of the interventions and/or what is the client's response to the interventions?

Example

1000 Diminished breath sounds in all lung fields with crackles in LLL. Not using incentive spirometer (IS). Stated he's "not sure how to use it." Temperature 99.6. Instructed how to use IS. Discussed the importance of deep breathing and coughing after surgery. Administered analgesic for c/o abdominal pain rating of 5/10. After pain relief (1/10), able to demonstrate correct use of

IS._____ S. Martin, RN
1400 Using IS each hour.
Lungs less diminished with fewer LLL crackles.
Temp 99._____ S. Martin, RN

2. SOAP

SOAP is an acronym for *s*ubjective data, *o*bjective data, *a*ssessment, and *p*lanning. The SOAP format originated with the problem-oriented medical record but is used increasingly in many different types of records. The acronyms SOAPIE and SOAPIER refer to formats that also include *i*mplementation, *e*valuation, and *r*evision. Many agencies use only the SOAP format. A more recent format is the APIE (*a*ssessment, *p*lan, *i*mplementation, and *e*valuation), which condenses the client data into fewer statements. In APIE, the assessment combines the nursing diagnosis; the plan combines the nursing actions with the expected outcomes; and the implementation and evaluation are the same. Figure 4–1 has examples of a nurse's progress notes using the SOAP, SOAPIER, and APIE formats.

3. Focus Charting (DAR)

Focus charting is intended to make the client and client concerns and strengths the focus of care. Three columns for recording are usually used: date and time, focus, and progress notes. The *focus* may be a condition, a nursing diagnosis, a behavior, a sign or symptom, an acute change in the client's condition, or a client strength. The progress notes are organized into (D) data, (A) action, and (R) response, referred to as DAR. The *data* category reflects the assessment phase of the nursing process and consists of observations of client status and behaviors, including data from flow sheets (e.g., vital signs, pupil reactivity). The nurse records both subjective and objective data in this section. The *action* category reflects planning and implementation and includes immediate and future nursing actions. It may also include any changes to the plan

Nursing Progress Notes

SOAP Format

6/6/07 1400 #5
S— "My skin is itchy on my back and arms, and it's been like this for a week."
O— Skin appears clear—no rash or irritation noted. Marks where client has scratched noted on left and right forearms. Allergic to Elastoplast but has not been in contact.
No previous history of pruritus.
A— Altered comfort (pruritus): cause unknown.

SOAPIER Format

6/6/07 1400 #5
S— Generalized pruritus
"My skin is itchy on my back and arms, and it's been like this for a week."
O— Skin appears clear—no rash or irritation noted. Marks where client has scratched noted on left and right forearms. Allergic to Elastoplast but has not been in contact.
No previous history of pruritus.
P— Altered comfort (pruritus): cause unknown.
P— Instruct not to scratch skin.
— Apply calamine lotion as necessary.
— Cut nails to avoid scratches.

APIE Format

6/6/07 1400
A— Generalized pruritus r/t unknown cause
States, "My skin is itchy on my back and arms, and it's been like this for a week." Skin appears clear. No rash or irritations noted. Marks where client has scratched noted on left and right forearms. Allergic to Elastoplast but has not been in contact. No previous history of pruritus.
P— Instruct not to scratch skin.
— Apply calamine lotion as necessary.
— Cut nails to avoid scratches.

P— Instructed not to scratch skin.

— Applied calamine lotion to back and arms at 1430 h.

— Cut fingernails to avoid scratches.

— Assess further to determine whether recurrence associated with specific drugs or foods.

— Refer to physician and pharmacist for assessment.
—*T. Ritchie, RN*

— Assess further to determine whether recurrence associated with specific drugs or foods.

— Refer to physician and pharmacist for assessment.

I— Instructed not to scratch skin.

Applied calamine lotion to back and arms at 1430 h.

Assisted to cut fingernails.

Notified physician and pharmacist of problem.

1600 E— States, "I'm still itchy. That lotion didn't help."

R— Remove calamine lotion and apply hydrocortisone cream as ordered. —*T. Ritchie, RN*

— Assess further to determine whether recurrence associated with specific drugs or foods.

— Refer to physician and pharmacist for assessment.

I— Instructed not to scratch skin.

Applied calamine lotion to back and arms at 1430 h.

Assisted to cut fingernails.

Notified physician and pharmacist of problem.

E— States, "I'm still itchy. That lotion didn't help."
—*T. Ritchie, RN*

Figure 4–1 ■ Examples of nursing progress notes using SOAP, SOAPIER, and APIE formats.

of care. The *response category* reflects the evaluation phase of the nursing process and describes the client's response to any nursing and medical care. See following example:

DAR Example

2/11/11 0900 Pain
D: Guarding abdominal incision. Facial grimacing. Rates pain at "8" on scale of 0–10.
A: Administered morphine sulfate 4 mg IV. 0930
R: Rates pain at "1." States willing to ambulate.

C. EVALUATION

Evaluation is the final phase of the nursing process, in which the nurse determines the client's progress toward goal/outcome achievement and the effectiveness of the nursing care plan.

The evaluation phase has five components:

- Collecting data related to the desired outcomes
- Comparing the data with desired outcomes
- Relating nursing activities to outcomes
- Drawing conclusions about problem status
- Continuing, modifying, or terminating the nursing care plan.

When determining whether a goal/outcome has been achieved, the nurse can draw one of three possible conclusions:

1. The goal was met; that is, the client response is the same as the desired outcome.
2. The goal was partially met; that is, either a short-term goal was achieved but the long-term goal was not, or the desired outcome was only partially attained.
3. The goal was not met.

When goals have been partially met or when goals have not been met, two conclusions may be drawn:

1. The care plan may need to be revised because the problem is only partially resolved. The revisions

may need to occur during assessing, diagnosing, or planning phases, as well as implementing.

2. The care plan does not need revision because the client merely needs more time to achieve the previously established goal(s). To make this decision, the nurse must assess why the goals are being only partially achieved, including whether the evaluation was conducted too soon.

UNIT 5

QUICK REFERENCE

A. Standard Precautions and Infection Control Strategies
B. Common Abbreviations and "Do Not Use" Abbreviations
C. Medical Terminology: Root Words, Prefixes, and Suffixes
D. Weight and Volume Conversions and Equivalents
E. Laboratory Values
F. Common Diagnostic Studies
G. Nursing Interventions for Endoscopic Examinations
H. Studies of the Gastrointestinal Tract
I. Studies of the Gallbladder and Bile Ducts
J. Radiographic Studies: Intravenous Pyelography, Angiography, Myelography
K. Key Information about Vitamins
L. Key Information about Minerals
M. Key Information about Trace Minerals

A. Standard Precautions and Infection Control Strategies

Recommended Infection Control Precautions in Hospitals

Standard Precautions

These precautions are used in the care of all clients regardless of their diagnosis or possible infection status:

- Designed for all clients
- Apply to (a) blood; (b) all body fluids, excretions, and secretions except sweat; (c) nonintact (broken) skin; and (d) mucous membranes
- Designed to reduce risk of transmission of microorganisms from recognized and unrecognized sources

1. Cleanse hands after contact with blood, body fluids, secretions, excretions, and contaminated objects regardless if gloves are worn.
   a. Cleanse hands immediately after removing gloves.
   b. Use a nonantimicrobial soap or alcohol-based gel for routine hand cleansing.
   c. Use an antimicrobial agent or an antiseptic agent for the control of specific outbreaks of infection.
2. Wear clean gloves when touching blood, body fluids, secretions, excretions, and contaminated items (e.g., soiled gowns).

a. Clean gloves can be unsterile unless they are intended to prevent the entrance of microorganisms into the body.

b. Remove gloves before touching noncontaminated items and surfaces.

c. Cleanse hands immediately after removing gloves.

3. Wear a mask, eye protection, or a face shield if splashes or sprays of blood, body fluids, secretions, or excretions can be expected.

4. Wear a clean, nonsterile water-resistent gown if client care is likely to result in splashes or sprays of blood, body fluids, secretions, or excretions. The gown is intended to protect clothing.

   a. Remove a soiled gown carefully to avoid the transfer of microorganisms to others (e.g., clients or other health care workers).

   b. Cleanse hands after removing gown.

5. Handle client care equipment that is soiled with blood, body fluids, secretions, or excretions carefully to prevent the transfer of microorganisms to others and to the environment.

   a. Make sure reusable equipment is cleaned and reprocessed correctly.

   b. Dispose of single-use equipment correctly.

6. Handle, transport, and process linen that is soiled with blood, body fluids, secretions, or excretions in a manner to prevent contamination of clothing and the transfer of microorganisms to others and to the environment.

7. Prevent injuries from used equipment such as scalpels or needles, and place them in puncture-resistant containers.

Transmission-Based Precautions

These precautions are used in addition to standard precautions for clients with known or suspected infection that is spread in one of three ways: by airborne or droplet transmission or by contact. The three types of transmission-based precautions may be used alone or in combination, but always *in addition to* standard precautions.

Airborne Precautions (for example: Rubeola, Tuberculosis, Varicella)

Use standard precautions as well as the following:

1. Place client in a private room that has negative air pressure, 6 to 12 air changes per hour, and discharge of air to the outside or a filtration system for the room air.
2. If a private room is not available, place client with another client who is infected with the same microorganism.
3. Wear a respiratory device (N95 respirator) when entering the room of a client who is known to have or suspected of having primary tuberculosis.
4. Susceptible people should not enter the room of a client who has rubella (measles) or varicella (chickenpox). If they must enter, they should wear a respirator.
5. Limit movement of client outside the room to essential purposes. Place a surgical mask on the client during transport.

Droplet Precautions (for example: Diphtheria, Pertussis, Mumps, Rubella)

Use standard precautions as well as the following:

1. Place client in a private room.
2. If a private room is not available, place client with another client who is infected with the same microorganism.
3. Wear a mask if working within 3 feet of the client.
4. Transport client outside of the room only when necessary and place a surgical mask on the client during transport.

Contact Precautions (for example: *C. difficile*, Hepatitis A, impetigo, drug-resistent *enterococci* and *Staphylococcus aureus*)

Use standard precautions as well as the following:

1. Place client in a private room.
2. If a private room is not available, place client with another client who is infected with the same microorganism.
3. Wear gloves as described in standard precautions.
   a. Change gloves after contact with infectious material.
   b. Remove gloves before leaving client's room.
   c. Cleanse hands immediately after removing gloves. Use an antimicrobial agent. Note: If the client is infected with *C. difficile*, do not use an alcohol-based hand rub because it is not effective on these spores. Use soap and water.
   d. After hand cleansing, do not touch possibly contaminated surfaces or items in the room.
4. Wear a gown (see Standard Precautions) when entering a room if there is a possibility of contact with infected surfaces or items or if the client is incontinent, has diarrhea, has a colostomy, or has wound drainage not contained by a dressing.
   a. Remove gown in the client's room.
   b. Make sure uniform does not contact possible contaminated surfaces.
5. Limit movement of client outside the room.
6. Dedicate the use of noncritical client care equipment to a single client or to clients with the same infecting microorganisms.

References

Siegel, J. D., Rhinehart, E., Jackson, M., Chiarello, L., & the Healthcare Infection Control Practices Advisory Committee. (2007). *2007 guidelines for isolation precautions: Preventing transmission of infectious agents in healthcare settings*. Retrieved from http://www.cdc.gov/hicpac/pdf/isolation/Isolation2007.pdf

Bloodborne Pathogens

Sometimes, despite the best practices, the nurse may be exposed to body substances likely to transmit bloodborne pathogens—those microorganisms carried in blood and body fluids that are capable of infecting other persons with serious and difficult-to-treat viral infections, namely hepatitis B virus, hepatitis C virus, and human immunodeficiency virus (HIV). Currently, all health care workers should be vaccinated against hepatitis B, but no vaccines are available for prevention of hepatitis C or HIV. The three major modes of transmission of infectious materials in the clinical setting are the following:

1. Puncture wounds from contaminated needles or other sharps
2. Skin contact, which allows infectious fluids to enter through wounds and broken or damaged skin
3. Mucous membrane contact, which allows infectious fluids to enter through mucous membranes of the eyes, mouth, and nose

It is critical that the nurse follow the next steps to ensure prompt evaluation and treatment, if indicated:

Steps to Follow after Exposure to Bloodborne Pathogens

- Report the incident immediately to appropriate personnel within the agency.
- Complete an injury report.
- Seek appropriate evaluation and follow-up. This includes the following:
  - Identification and documentation of the source individual when feasible and legal

  - Testing of the source for hepatitis B, hepatitis C, and HIV when feasible and consent is given
  - Making results of the test available to the source individual's health care provider
  - Testing of blood of exposed nurse (with consent) for hepatitis B, hepatitis C, and HIV antibodies
  - Postexposure prophylaxis if medically indicated
  - Medical and psychological counseling regarding personal risk of infection or risk of infecting others
- For a puncture/laceration
  - Allow some bleeding to drain the site but do not squeeze the tissues
  - Wash/clean the area with soap and water
  - Initiate first aid and seek treatment if indicated
- For a mucous membrane exposure (eyes, nose, mouth), perform saline or water flush for 5 to 10 minutes.

Postexposure Prophylaxis

Human Immunodeficiency Virus

Treatment should be started as soon as possible, preferably within hours after exposure. Treatment may be less effective when started more than 24 hours after exposure. Starting treatment after a longer period (e.g., 1 week) should be considered for high-risk exposures previously untreated.

- For high-risk exposure (high blood volume *and* source with a high HIV titer): three-drug treatment is recommended.
- For increased-risk exposure (high blood volume *or* source with a high HIV titer): three-drug treatment is recommended.
- For low-risk exposure (*neither* high blood volume *nor* source with a high HIV titer): two-drug treatment is considered.

- Drug prophylaxis is for 4 weeks. If the source is determined to be HIV negative, prophylaxis should be discontinued.
- Drug regimens vary and new drugs and regimens are continuously being developed.
- HIV antibody tests done shortly after exposure (baseline), and 6 weeks, 3 months, and 6 months afterward.

Hepatitis B

- Testing for antibodies to hepatitis B surface antigen (anti-HBs), administering booster dose or immune globulin if not immune

Hepatitis C

- Testing for antibodies to hepatitis C surface antigen (Anti-HCV) and for alanine aminotransferase (ALT) at baseline and 4 to 6 months after exposure

Infection Control Strategies

- Use strict aseptic technique when performing any invasive procedure (e.g., inserting an intravenous needle or catheter, suctioning an airway, and inserting a urinary catheter).
- Handle needles and syringes carefully to avoid needle stick injuries.
- Change intravenous tubing and solution containers according to agency policy (e.g., every 48 to 72 hours).
- Check all sterile supplies for expiration date and intact packaging.
- Prevent urinary infections by maintaining a closed urinary drainage system with a downhill flow of urine; do not irrigate a catheter unless ordered to do so; provide regular catheter care; and keep the drainage bag and spout off the floor.
- Implement measures to prevent impaired skin integrity and to prevent accumulation of secretions in the lungs (e.g., encourage the client to move, cough, and breathe deeply at least every 2 hours).

Preventing Infections in the Home

The nurse teaches the client and family members to do the following:

- Wash hands before handling foods, before eating, after toileting, before and after any required home care treatment, and after touching any body substances (e.g., wound drainage).
- Keep fingernails short, clean, and well-manicured to eliminate rough edges or hangnails, which can harbor microorganisms.
- Do not share personal care items: toothbrush, washcloths, and towels.
- Wash raw fruits and vegetables before eating them.
- Refrigerate all opened and nonpackaged foods.
- Clean used equipment (e.g., emesis basin) with soap and water, and disinfect with a chlorine bleach solution.
- Place contaminated dressings and other disposable items containing body fluids in moisture-proof plastic bags.
- Put used needles in a puncture-resistant container with a screw-top lid. Label so as not to discard in the garbage.
- Clean obviously soiled linen separately from other laundry. Rinse in cold water, wash in hot water if possible, and add a cup of bleach or Lysol to the wash.
- Avoid coughing, sneezing, or breathing directly on others. Cover the mouth and nose to prevent the transmission of airborne microorganisms.
- Be aware of any signs or symptoms of an infection, and report these immediately to the health care provider.
- Maintain a sufficient fluid intake to promote urine production and output. This helps flush the bladder and urethra of microorganisms.

B. Common Abbreviations and "Do Not Use" Abbreviations

Common Abbreviations

Abbreviation	Term
abd	abdomen
ABO	the main blood group system
ac	before meals (ante cibum)
ADL	activities of daily living
ad lib	as desired (ad libitum)
adm	admitted or admission
AM	morning (ante meridiem)
amb	ambulatory
amt	amount
approx	approximately (about)
bid	twice daily (bis in die)
BM (bm)	bowel movement
BP	blood pressure
BR	bed rest
BRP	bathroom privileges
c̄	with
C	Celsius (centigrade)
CBC	complete blood count
c/o	complains of
DAT	diet as tolerated
DNR	do not resuscitate
drsg	dressing
Dx	diagnosis
ECG (EKG)	electrocardiogram
F	Fahrenheit
fld	fluid

Abbreviation	Term
GI	gastrointestinal
gtt	drops (guttae)
h (hr)	hour (hora)
H_2O	water
I & O	intake and output
IV	intravenous
LMP	last menstrual period
(L)	left
meds	medications
mL (ml)	milliliter
mod	moderate
neg	negative
Ø	none
#	number
NPO (NBM)	nothing by mouth (nil per os)
NS (N/S)	normal saline
O_2	oxygen
OD	right eye (oculus dexter); overdose
OOB	out of bed
OS	left eye (oculus sinister)
pc	after meals (post cibum)
PE (PX)	physical examination
per	by or through
PM	afternoon (post meridiem)
po	by mouth (per os)
postop	postoperative(ly)
preop	preoperative(ly)
prep	preparation
prn	when necessary (pro re nata)
qid	four times a day (quater in die)
(R)	right
$\bar{s}$	without (sine)
stat	at once, immediately (statim)
tid	three times a day (ter in die)
TO	telephone order
TPR	temperature, pulse, respirations
VO	verbal order
VS (vs)	vital signs
WNL	within normal limits
wt	weight

(continued)

B. Common Abbreviations and "Do Not Use" Abbreviations (*continued*)

"Do Not Use" List Do Not Use	Potential Problem	Use Instead
U (unit)	Mistaken as 9 (zero), the number "4" (four), or cc	Write "unit"
IU (for international unit)	Mistaken as IV (intravenous) or the number 10 (ten)	Write "international unit"
Q.D., Q.O.D (Latin abbreviation for "once daily" and "every other day")	Mistaken for each other. The period after the Q can be mistaken for an "I" and the "O" can be mistaken for "I".	Write "daily" and "every other day"
Trailing zero (X.0 mg) (Note: prohibited only for medication-related notations); lack of leading zero (.X mg)	Decimal point is missed	Never write a zero by itself after a decimal point (X mg), and always use a zero before a decimal point (0.X mg)
MS, MSO_4, and $MgSO_4$	Confused for one another. Can mean morphine sulfate or magnesium sulfate	Write "morphine sulfate" or "magnesium sulfate"
The following items will be reviewed annually for possible inclusion on the "Do Not Use" list:		
≧ (greater than) ≦ (less than)	Misinterpreted as the number "7" (seven) or the letter "L" Confused for one another	Write "greater than" Write "less than"
Abbreviations for drug names	Misinterpreted due to similar abbreviations for multiple drugs	Write drug names in full
Apothecary units	Unfamiliar to many practitioners Confused with metric units	Use metric units

Do Not Use	Potential Problem	Use Instead
@	Mistaken for the number "2" (two)	Write "at"
c.c. (for cubic centimeter)	Mistaken for U (units) when poorly written	Write "mL" or "milliliters" ("mL" is preferred)
µg (for microgram)	Mistaken for mg (milligrams) resulting in one thousand-fold dosing overdose	Write "mcg" or "micrograms"
Others to Consider		
TIW (three times a week)	Has been misinterpreted as "two times a week" or "three times a day" resulting in misdosing	Write "three times weekly"
AS (left ear) AD (right ear) AU (both ears)	Mistaken for OS (left eye), OD (either "overdose" or "optic density"), and OU ("each eye" or "both eyes")	Write "left ear," "right ear," or "both ears," as appropriate
HS	Has been used to indicate "half strength" and "bedtime" or "hour of sleep"	Write out "half strength" or "at bedtime," as appropriate
SC and SQ (subcutaneous)	Have been read as "SL" (sublingual) and as "5 every hour"	Write "subq" or "subcutaneous"
D/C	Can mean either "discharge" or "discontinue"	Write "discharge" or "discontinue" as appropriate

C. Medical Terminology: Root Words, Prefixes, and Suffixes

Word Element	Meaning
Root Words	
Circulatory System	
cardio	heart
angio, vaso	vessel
hem, hema, hemato	blood
vena, phlebo	vein
arteria	artery
lympho	lymph
thrombo	clot (of blood)
embolus	moving clot
Digestive System	
bucca	cheek
os, stomato	mouth
gingiva	gum
glossa	tongue
pharyngo	pharynx
esophago	esophagus
gastro	stomach
hepato	liver
cholecyst	gallbladder
pancreas	pancreas
entero	intestines
duodeno	duodenum
jejuno	jejunum
ileo	ileum
caeco	cecum
appendeco	appendix
colo	colon

Word Element	Meaning
recto	rectum
ano, procto	anus
Skeletal System	
skeleto	skeleton
Respiratory System	
naso, rhino	nose
tonsillo	tonsil
laryngo	larynx
tracheo	trachea
bronchus, broncho	bronchus (pl. bronchi)
pulmo, pneuma, pneum	lung (sac with air)
Nervous System	
neuro	nerve
cerebrum	brain
oculo, ophthalmo	eye
oto	ear
psych, psycho	mind
Urinary System	
urethro	urethra
cysto	bladder
uretero	ureter
reni, reno, nephro	kidney
pyleo	pelvis of kidney
uro	urine
Female Reproductive System	
vulvo	vulva
perineo	perineum
labio	labium (pl. labia)
vagino, colpo	vagina
cervico	cervix
utero	womb; uterus
tubo, salpingo	fallopian tube
ovario, oophoro	ovary
Male Reproductive System	
orchido	testes
Regions of the Body	
crani, cephalo	head
cervico, tracheo	neck
thoraco	chest

(continued)

C. Medical Terminology (*Continued*)

Word Element	Meaning
abdomino	abdomen
dorsum	back
Tissues	
cutis, dermato	skin
lipo	fat
musculo, myo	muscle
osteo	bone
myelo	marrow
chondro	cartilage
Miscellaneous	
cyto	cell
genetic	formation, origin
gram	tracing or mark
graph	writing, description
kinesis	motion
meter	measure
oligo	small, few
phobia	fear
photo	light
pyo	pus
scope	instrument for visual examination
roentgen	x-ray
lapar	flank; through the abdominal wall
Prefixes	
a, an, ar	without or not
ab	away from
acro	extremities
ad	toward, to
adeno	glandular
aero	air
ambi	around, on both sides
amyl	starch
ante	before, forward
anti	against, counteracting
bi	double
bili	bile
bio	life
bis	two
brachio	arm

Word Element	Meaning
brady	slow
broncho	bronchus (pl. bronchi)
cardio	heart
cervico	neck
chole	gall or bile
cholecysto	gallbladder
circum	around
co	together
contra	against, opposite
costo	ribs
cyto	cell
cysto	bladder
demi	half
derma	skin
dis	from
dorso	back
dys	abnormal, difficult
electro	electric
en	into, in, within
encephal	brain
entero	intestine
equi	equal
eryth	red
ex	out, out of, away from
extra	outside of, in addition to
ferro	iron
fibro	fiber
fore	before, in front of
gastro	stomach
glosso	tongue
glyco	sugar
hemi	half
hemo	blood
hepa, hepato	liver
histo	tissue
homo	same
hydro	water
hygro	moisture
hyper	too much, high

(continued)

C. Medical Terminology (*Continued*)

Word Element	Meaning
hypo	under, decreased
hyster	uterus
ileo	ileum
in	in, within, into
inter	between
intra	within
intro	in, within, into
juxta	near, close to
laryngo	larynx
latero	side
lapar	abdomen
leuk	white
macro	large, big
mal	bad, poor
mast	breast
medio	middle
mega, megalo	large, great
meno	menses
mono	single
multi	many
myelo	bone marrow, spinal cord
myo	muscle
neo	new
nephro	kidney
neuro	nerve
nitro	nitrogen
noct	night
non	not
ob	against, in front of
oculo	eye
odonto	tooth
ophthalmo	eye
ortho	straight, normal
os	mouth, bone
osteo	bone
oto	ear
pan	all
para	beside, accessory to
path	disease
ped	child, foot

Word Element	Meaning
per	by, through
peri	around
pharyngo	pharynx
phlebo	vein
photo	light
phren	diaphragm, mind
pneumo	air, lungs
pod	foot
poly	many, much
post	after
pre	before
proct	rectum
pseudo	false
psych	mind
pyel	pelvis of the kidney
pyo	pus
pyro	fever, heat
quadri	four
radio	radiation
re	back, again
reno	kidney
retro	backward
rhin	nose
sacro	sacrum
salpingo	fallopian tube
sarco	flesh
sclero	hard, hardening
semi	half
sex	six
skeleto	skeleton
steno	narrowing, constriction
sub	under
super	above, excess
supra	above
syn	together
tachy	fast
thyro	thyroid, gland
trache	trachea
trans	across, over
tri	three

(continued)

C. Medical Terminology (*Continued*)

Word Element	Meaning
ultra	beyond
un	not, back, reversal
uni	one
uretero	ureter
urethro	urethra
uro	urine, urinary organs
vaso	vessel
Suffixes	
able	able to
algia	pain
cele	tumor, swelling
centesis	surgical puncture to remove fluid
cide	killing, destructive
cule	little
cyte	cell
ectasia	dilating, stretching
ectomy	excision, surgical removal of
emia	blood
esis	action
form	shaped like
genesis, genetic	formation, origin
gram	tracing, mark
graph	writing
ism	condition
itis	inflammation
ize	to treat
lith	stone, calculus
lithiasis	presence of stones
lysis	disintegration
megaly	enlargement
meter	instrument that measures
oid	likeness, resemblance
oma	tumor
opathy	disease of
orrhaphy	surgical repair
osis	disease, condition of
ostomy	to form an opening or outlet
otomy	to incise
pexy	fixation

Word Element	Meaning
phage	ingesting
phobia	fear
plasty	plastic surgery
plegia	paralysis
rhage	to burst forth
rhea	excessive discharge
rhexis	rupture
scope	lighted instrument for visual examination
scopy	to examine visually
stomy	to form an opening
tomy	incision into
uria	urine

D. Weight and Volume Conversions and Equivalents

Prefix	Abbreviations	Numerical	Value
Basic Metric Units			
kilo	k	1000	one thousand
hecto	h	100	one hundred
deka	dk	10	ten
deci	d	0.1	one-tenth
centi	c	0.01	one-hundredth
milli	M	0.001	one-thousandth
micro	mc, μ	0.000001	one-millionth

Metric Weight Equivalents

1 kg (kilogram)	= 1000 g (grams)
1 g (gram)	= 1000 mg (milligrams)
1 mg (milligram)	= 1000 mcg, μg (micrograms)

Approximate Weight Equivalents: Metric and Apothecaries' Systems

Metric	Apothecaries'
0.1 mg	1/600 grain (gr)
0.6 mg	1/100 grain
1 mg	1/60 grain
4 mg	1/15 grain
6 mg	1/10 grain
10 mg	1/6 grain
15 mg	1/4 grain
30 mg	1/2 grain
60 mg	1 grain
500 mg (0.5 g)	7 1/2 grains
600 mg (0.6 g)	10 grains
1 g (1000 mg)	15 grains

2 g	30 grains
4 g	60 grains (1 dram)
7.5 g	120 grains (2 drams)
30 g	1 ounce (8 drams)
1000 g	2.2 pounds (1 kilogram)

Approximate Volume Equivalents: Metric, Apothecaries', and Household Systems

Metric	Apothecaries'	Household
0.06 mL	1 minim (m)	1 drop (gt)
0.3 mL	5 minims	5 drops (gtt)
0.6 mL	10 minims	10 drops (gtt)
1 mL (1 cubic cm)	15 minims	15 drops (gtt)
2 mL	30 minims	30 drops (gtt)
3 mL	45 minims	45 drops (gtt)
5 mL	60 minims	60 drops
	(1 fluid dram [ʒ])	(1 teaspoon [tsp])
8 mL	2 fluid drams	2 teaspoons
15 mL	4 fluid drams	3 teaspoons
		(1 tablespoon)
30 mL	8 fluid drams	2 tablespoons
	(1 fluid ounce [℥])	
60 mL	2 fluid ounces	
90 mL	3 fluid ounces	
200 mL	6 fluid ounces	1 teacup
250 mL	8 fluid ounces	1 large glass
500 mL	16 fluid ounces	1 pint
	(1 pint [pt])	
1000 mL (1 liter)	2 pints	1 quart
	(1 quart [qt])	
4000 mL	4 quarts	
1 gallon (gal)		

E. Laboratory Values

The ranges for normal values may vary from laboratory to laboratory; therefore, always check with each agency for its own normal range and for the particular testing method, and, if indicated, for the population for which the set of values is described. All values should be interpreted within the context of the client's health status. Refer to Chapter 52 of *Fundamentals of Nursing* for a thorough discussion of fluids, electrolytes, and acid–base balance.

Table A Complete Blood Count with Clinical Implications

Component	Normal Findings (Adult)	Possible Causes of Abnormal Findings	
		Increased	Decreased
Red blood cell (RBC) count The number of RBCs per cubic millimeter (mm^3).	Men: 4.6–6.0 million/mm^3 Women: 4.0–5.0 million/mm^3	Primary polycythemia (e.g., polycythemia vera) Secondary polycythemia or erythrocytosis—usually caused by oxygen need (e.g., chronic lung disease, congenital heart defects)	Abnormal loss of erythrocytes Abnormal destruction of erythrocytes Lack of needed elements or hormones for erythrocyte production Bone marrow suppression Lead poisoning Thalassemia
Hemoglobin (Hgb) Composed of a pigment (heme), which contains iron, and a protein (globin).	Men: 13.5–18 g/dL Women: 12–15 g/dL Anemia is classified when the hemoglobin level falls below 10.5 g/dL.	Polycythemia	Blood loss Hemolytic anemia Bone marrow suppression Sickle cell anemia

(*continued*)

Table A Complete Blood Count with Clinical Implications (*Continued*)

Component	Normal Findings (Adult)	Possible Causes of Abnormal Findings	
		Increased	Decreased
Hematocrit (Hct)			
The hematocrit or packed cell volume (Hct, PCV, or crit) is a fast way to determine the percentage of RBCs in the plasma. The Hct is reported as a percentage because it is the proportion of RBCs to the plasma.	Men: 40–54% Women: 36–46%	Dehydration Burns Hypovolemia	Blood loss Overhydration Dietary deficiency Anemia
RBC indices			
Mean corpuscular volume (MCV) The mean or average size of the individual RBC.	Men: 80–98 μm^3 Women: 78–102 μm^3	Liver disease Alcoholism Pernicious anemia	Microcytic iron deficiency anemia Lead poisoning Iron deficiency anemia
Mean corpuscular hemoglobin (MCH) Amount of Hgb present in one cell.	25–35 pg	Rarely seen	
Mean corpuscular hemoglobin concentration (MCHC) The proportion of each cell occupied by Hgb.	31–37%	Rarely seen	Iron deficiency anemia

White blood cell (WBC) count Count of the total number of WBCs in a cubic millimeter of blood.	4,500–11,000/mm^3	Leukocytosis Infection	Leukopenia Autoimmune disease
Differential count: The proportion of each of the five types of WBCs in a sample of 100 WBCs.			
Neutrophils	50–70%	Stress Acute infection	Viral diseases Some drugs (e.g., chemotherapy, antibiotics such as nafcillin, penicillin, and cephalosporins) Radiation therapy
Lymphocytes	25–45%	Viral infection Mononucleosis Tuberculosis Chronic bacterial infections Lymphocytic leukemia	Adrenal corticosteroids and other immunosuppressive drugs Autoimmune diseases (e.g., lupus erythematosus) Severe malnutrition

(*continued*)

Table A Complete Blood Count with Clinical Implications (*Continued*)

Component	Normal Findings (Adult)	Possible Causes of Abnormal Findings	
		Increased	Decreased
Monocytes	4–6%	Chronic inflammatory disorders Tuberculosis Protozoan infections (e.g., malaria, Rocky Mountain spotted fever) Chronic ulcerative colitis	Drug therapy: prednisone
Eosinophils	1–3%	Allergic reactions (e.g., asthma, hay fever, or hypersensitivity to a drug) Parasitic infestations (e.g., round worms)	Corticosteroid therapy
Basophils	0.4–1.0%	Leukemia	Acute allergic reaction Corticosteroids Acute infections

Platelet count Platelets are fragments of cytoplasm that function in blood coagulation.	150,000–350,000/mm^3	Malignant tumors Polycythemia vera	Idiopathic (unknown cause) Thrombocytopenic purpura Viral infections AIDS Systemic lupus erythematosus Chemotherapy drugs Some types of anemias

From *Laboratory and Diagnostic Tests with Nursing Implications*, 6th ed. (pp. 212–214; 320–321; 345–346; 400–403), by J. Kee, 2009. Upper Saddle River, NJ: Pearson Education.

Table B. Common Blood Chemistry Tests with Clinical Implications

Test	Normal Findings (Adult)	Significance	Possible Causes of Increased	Possible Causes of Decreased
Liver Function Tests				
ALT (alanine amino transferase), formerly known as serum pyretic transaminase (SGPT)	Men: 10–55 unit/L Women: 7–30 unit/L	Marker of hepatic injury; more specific of liver damage than AST	Hepatitis, infectious mononucleosis, acute pancreatitis, acute myocardial infarction, heart failure	Not clinically significant
AST (aspartate amino transferase) formerly known as serum glutamic-oxaloacetic transaminase (SGOT)	Men: 10–40 unit/L Women: 9–25 unit/L	Found in heart, liver, and skeletal muscle. Can also be used to indicate liver injury	Liver diseases (e.g., hepatitis, alcoholism, drug toxicity), acute myocardial infarction, anemias, skeletal muscle diseases	Chronic renal dialysis, vitamin B_6 deficiency
Albumin	Adults: 3.5–4.8 g/dL or 35–48 g/L Panic value: $<$1.5 g/dL	Is a protein produced by the liver	No pathology causes the liver to produce more albumin. An increased level reflects dehydration	Chronic liver dysfunction, AIDS, severe burns, malnutrition, renal disease, acute and chronic infections

Alkaline phosphatase	Adults: 25–100 unit/L	Found in the tissues of the liver, bone, intestine, kidney, and placenta. Used as an index of liver and bone disease when correlated with other clinical findings	Liver disease, bone disease, hyperparathyroidism, myocardial infarction, chronic renal failure, heart failure	Malnutrition, pernicious anemia and severe anemias, hypothyroidism, magnesium and zinc deficiency (nutritional)
Ammonia	Adults: 15–45 mcg/dl	The liver converts ammonia, a by-product of protein metabolism, into urea which is excreted by the kidneys	Liver disease, cirrhosis, Reye's syndrome, GI hemorrhage	Renal failure
Bilirubin	Adults: Total: 0.3–1.0 mg/dL Direct: 0.0–0.2 mg/dL Indirect: 0.1–1/0 mg/dL Panic value: >12 mg/dL	Results from the breakdown of hemoglobin in the red blood cells; removed from the body by the liver, which excretes it into the bile	Total: hepatitis, obstruction of the common bile or hepatic ducts, pernicious anemia, sickle cell anemia Direct: cancer of the head of the pancreas, choledocholithiasis Indirect: hemolytic anemias, drug toxicity, transfusion reaction	Not clinically significant

(*continued*)

Table B Common Blood Chemistry Tests with Clinical Implications (*Continued*)

Test	Normal Findings (Adult)	Significance	Possible Causes of Increased	Possible Causes of Decreased
GGT (gamma-glutamyl transferase)	Men: 1–94 unit/L Women: 1–70 unit/L	Found primarily in the liver, kidney, prostate, and spleen. Is more specific for the hepatobiliary system.	Liver disease, alcohol abuse	Not clinically significant
Prothrombin	11–13 seconds Critical value: >20 seconds for non-anticoagulated persons	A protein produced by the liver for clotting of blood	Liver disease, damage, vitamin K deficiency, obstruction of common bile duct, deficiency of factors II, V, VII, or X	Thrombophlebitis, malignant tumor
Cardiac Markers				
CK (creatine kinase)	Total: Men: 38–174 unit/L Women: 26–140 unit/L Isoenzymes: MM (CK_3): 96–100% MB (CK_2): 0–6% BB (CK_1): 0%	An enzyme found in the heart and skeletal muscles. Has three isoenzymes: MM or CK_3, MB or CK_2, and BB or CK_1	Total: acute myocardial infarction (MI), myocarditis, after open heart surgery, acute cerebrovascular disease, muscular dystrophy, chronic alcoholism CK isoenzymes: MB (CK_2): myocardial infarct, myocardial ischemia, angina pectoris	Not clinically significant

Myoglobin	5–70 ng/mL	After an MI, serum levels of myoglobin rise in 2–4 hours, making it an early marker for muscle damage in MI	Myocardial infarction, angina, other muscle injury (e.g., trauma), renal failure, rhabdomyolysis	Rheumatoid arthritis, myasthenia gravis
Troponin I Troponin T	Troponin I: <0.35 ng/mL Critical value: >1.5 ng/mL Troponin T: <0.2 ng/mL	Cardiac troponin is highly concentrated in the heart muscle. This test is used in the early diagnosis of MI. After an MI, troponin I begins to increase in 4–6 hours and remains elevated for 5–7 days Troponin T begins to increase in 3–4 hours and remains elevated for 10–14 days	Troponin I: small infarct, myocardial injury Troponin T: Acute MI, unstable angina, myocarditis	Not clinically significant

(*continued*)

Table B Common Blood Chemistry Tests with Clinical Implications (*Continued*)

Test	Normal Findings (Adult)	Significance	Possible Causes of Increased	Possible Causes of Decreased
BNP (Brain Natriuretic Peptide or B-type natriuretic peptide)	<100 pg/mL or <100 ng/L	A hormone produced by the ventricles of the heart; is a marker of ventricular systolic and diastolic dysfunction. This test is useful in diagnosing and guiding treatment of heart failure	Heart failure, symptomatic cardiac volume overload, paroxysmal atrial tachycardia	Not clinically significant
Lipoprotein Profile				
Cholesterol	Adults: Desirable: <200 mg/dL	This test is an important screening test for heart disease	Type II familial hypercholesterolemia, biliary cirrhosis, chronic renal failure, poorly controlled diabetes mellitus, alcoholism, diet high in cholesterol and fats	Severe hepatocellular disease, hyperthyroidism, malnutrition, chronic anemias, severe burns

HDL-C (high-density lipoprotein cholesterol)	Men: 35–65 mg/dL Women: 35–80 mg/dL	A class of lipoproteins produced by the liver and intestines; the "good" cholesterol	HDL excess, chronic liver disease, long-term aerobic or vigorous exercise	Familial hypolipoproteinemia, hypertriglyceridemia (familial), poorly controlled diabetes mellitus, chronic renal failure
LDL (low-density lipoprotein)	Adults: Desirable: <130 mg/dL	Up to 70% of the total serum cholesterol is present in LDL; the "bad" cholesterol	Familial type 2 hyperlipidemia Secondary causes can include diet high in cholesterol and saturated fat, nephritic syndrome, multiple myeloma, diabetes mellitus, chronic renal failure	Hypolipoproteinemia, hyperthyroidism, chronic anemias, severe hepatocellular disease
Triglycerides	Desirable: <150 mg/dL	This test evaluates suspected atherosclerosis and measures the body's ability to metabolize fat	Hyperlipoproteinemia, liver disease, renal disease, hypothyroidism, pancreatitis, myocardial infarction	Malnutrition, hyperthyroidism, brain infarction, chronic obstructive lung disease

Table C Serum Electrolytes

Test	Normal Findings (Adult)	Possible Causes of Increased	Possible Causes of Decreased
Sodium	135–145 mEq/L	Cushing's syndrome Dehydration Diabetes insipidus Excessive intravenous sodium Insufficient water intake Impaired renal function	Severe burns Addison's disease Diabetic ketoacidosis Diuretic therapy Excessive gastrointestinal tract loss Water intoxication
Potassium	3.5–5.0 mEq/L	Acidosis Diabetic ketoacidosis Hypoaldosteronism Massive crushing tissue destruction Renal failure Use of potassium-sparing diuretics	Alkalosis Cushing's syndrome Diarrhea (severe) Diuretic therapy Gastrointestinal fistula Pyloric obstruction Starvation Vomiting Alcoholism Burns

Chloride	95–105 mEq/L	Cushing's syndrome Dehydration Hypernatremia Metabolic acidosis Respiratory alkalosis Kidney dysfunction	Overhydration Addison's disease Burns (severe) Diarrhea Diuretic use Metabolic alkalosis Chronic respiratory acidosis Vomiting Gastric suctioning
Calcium (total)	4.5–5.5 mEq/L or 8.5–10.5 mg/ dL	Total calcium: Hyperparathyroidism Cancers Hyperthyroidism Prolonged immobility Paget's disease	Total calcium: Reduced albumin Hypoparathyroidism Alkalosis Acute pancreatitis Vitamin D deficiency
Calcium (ionized)	56% of total calcium (2.5 mEq/L or 4.0–5.0 mg/dL)	Ionized calcium: Hypoparathyroidism Excess vitamin D intake	Ionized calcium: Acute pancreatitis Diabetic acidosis Hyperventilation Vitamin D deficiency

(*Continued*)

Table C Serum Electrolytes (*Continued*)

Test	Normal Findings (Adult)	Possible Causes of Increased	Possible Causes of Decreased
Magnesium	1.5–2.5 mEq/L or 2.5–4.5 mg/dL	Addison's disease Dehydration Diabetic ketoacidosis Excessive use of magnesium-containing antacids Hypothyroidism Renal disorders	Hemodialysis Blood transfusions Chronic alcoholism Chronic renal disease Hypoparathyroidism Hyperthyroidism Severe burns
Phosphate (phosphorus)	1.8–2.6 mEq/L or 2.5–4.5 mg/dL	Hypocalcemia Hypoparathyroidism Renal disease Skeletal disease Liver disease Bone metastasis	Malabsorption Chronic alcoholism Diabetes mellitus Hypercalcemia Hyperparathyroidism Vitamin D deficiency
Serum osmolality	280–300 mOsm/kg water	Hypernatremia Dehydration Hyperglycemia Chronic renal disease Diabetes insipidus	Malnutrition Hyponatremia Fluid volume excess Syndrome of inappropriate antidi uretic hormone secretion (SIADH)

Table D Arterial Blood Gases

Test	Normal Findings (Adult)	Possible Causes of Increased	Possible Causes of Decreased
pH	7.35–7.45	Alkalosis (metabolic and respiratory)	Acidosis (metabolic and respiratory)
PaO_2	80–100 mm Hg	Administration of high concentration of oxygen	Chronic lung disease Anemia
$PaCO_2$	35–45 mm Hg	Respiratory acidosis or compensated metabolic alkalosis	Respiratory alkalosis or compensated metabolic acidosis
HCO_3	22–26 mEq/L	Metabolic alkalosis	Metabolic acidosis
Base excess	−2 to +2 mEq/L	Metabolic alkalosis	Metabolic acidosis
Oxygen saturation	95–98%	Polycythemia	Anemia Cardiac decompensation Respiratory disorders

Table E Urine Chemistry

Test	Specimen	Normal Values: Conventional Units	Normal Values: SI Units	Possible Etiologies: Higher	Possible Etiologies: Lower
Bilirubin	Random	Negative	Negative	Cirrhosis; gallstone; hepatic obstruction; hepatitis	—
Calcium	24h	100–300 mg/day	2.5–7.5 mmol/day	Bone metastases; hyperparathyroidism; breast and bladder cancers	Calcium and vitamin D malabsorption; hypoparathyroidism; renal disease
Creatinine	24h			Acromegaly; diabetes mellitus; hyperthyroidism	Heart failure; renal disease; shock; hypothyroidism
Male		0.8–1.8 g/day	7.1–17.7 mmol/day		
Female		0.6–1.6 g/day	5.3–15.9 mmol/day		
Creatinine clearance	24h			Exercise; pregnancy; high cardiac output syndromes	Impaired kidney function; heart failure; cirrhosis; shock
Male		70–150 mL/min	1.42–2.25 mL/sec		
Female		85–132 mL/min	1.42–2.25 mL/sec		
Glucose	Random	Negative	Negative	Cushing's syndrome; diabetes mellitus; pregnancy	—

Hemoglobin	Random	Negative	Negative	Hematuria: trauma to kidneys; glomerulonephritis; hemolytic transfusion reaction; urinary tract infections; urinary calculi; hemoglobinuria; burns; transfusion reaction; sickle cell anemia	—
Ketone bodies	Random dip stick	Negative	Negative	Diabetes (uncontrolled); fasting; high-protein diet; starvation; pregnancy	—
pH	Random	4.6–8.0	4.6–8.0	Alkalosis; chronicrenal failure; diuretic use; gastric suction; salicylate intoxica tion; urinary tract infection; vegetable diet; vomiting	Acidosis; dehydration; starvation; urinary tract infections
Protein (dipstick)	Random	Negative	Negative	Congestive heart failure; glomerulosclero sis; lupus erythematosus; multiple myeloma; nephrotic syndrome	—
Specific gravity	Random	1.010–1.025	1.010–1.025	Albuminuria; dehydration; diarrhea; glycosuria; presence of contrast medium; vomiting	Diabetes insipidus; overhydration; renal disease
Uric acid	24h	250–750 mg/day	1.5–4.5 mmol/day	Gout; hepatic disease; sickle cell anemia	Chronic glomerulonephritis; lead toxicity; nephritis

Reference

Kee, J. (2009). *Laboratory and diagnostic tests with nursing implications* (6th ed.). Upper Saddle River, NJ: Pearson Education.

F. Common Diagnostic Studies

Test	Purpose
Blood	
Complete blood count (CBC)	To determine hemoglobin (Hgb), hematocrit (Hct), and erythrocyte, or red blood cell (RBC) count and assess the blood's ability to carry oxygen; to determine the leukocyte, or white blood cell (WBC) count, which signals infection when elevated.
Serum electrolytes (Na^+, K^+, Mg^{2+}, Ca^{2+}, H^+)	To determine electrolyte and acid–base imbalances.
Arterial blood gas (ABG) analysis	To determine the adequacy of alveolar gas exchange and evaluate the ability of the lungs and kidneys to maintain the acid–base balance of the body fluids. ABGs include pH, P_{CO_2}, bicarbonate, P_{O_2} and oxygen saturation, and base excess.
Fasting blood sugar (FBS) test	To detect presence of glucose in the blood, which may indicate metabolic disorders (e.g., diabetes mellitus).
Glucose tolerance test (GTT)	To determine ability to tolerate a standard glucose load (insulin response) without spillage over into the urine.
Blood urea nitrogen (BUN) or creatinine	To assess urinary excretion.
Sputum	
Sputum culture and sensitivity test	To determine the presence of pathogenic bacteria and bacterial sensitivity to various antibiotics.
Acid-fast bacilli (AFB) test	To determine the presence of acid-fast bacilli, indicating, for example, active tuberculosis.
Cytologic tests	To determine the presence of abnormal or malignant cells.

Test	Purpose
Urine	
Urinalysis (UA)	To detect urinary tract infections and glucose in the urine.
Urine culture and sensitivity test	To determine the presence of pathogenic bacteria and bacterial sensitivity to various antibiotics.
Stool	
Guaiac test	To determine the presence of occult blood and bleeding in the gastrointestinal tract.
Ova and parasite tests (O & P)	To determine the presence of a parasitic infection of the intestine.
Radiologic	
Chest roentgenogram (CXR)	To identify lung disease and heart size and location.
Upper gastrointestinal (UGI) test	To identify lesions in the esophagus, stomach, and duodenum after barium, a contrast medium, is swallowed.
Lower gastrointestinal (LGI) test	To identify lesions of the large bowel after a barium enema.
Scan of the head, chest, bone, or entire body	A noninvasive x-ray procedure that distinguishes minor differences in the radiodensity of soft tissues (e.g., a tumor in liver tissue).
Other	
Electrocardiogram (ECG or EKG)	To determine the presence of cardiac disease.
Exercise stress test	To determine the client's ability to obtain and maintain maximum heart rate of 85% for pre dicted age and sex with no cardiac symptoms or ECG (EKG) change.
Tuberculin (TB) skin test	To detect tuberculosis infection; however, does not indicate whether the infection is active or dormant.

G. Nursing Interventions for Endoscopic Examinations

Examination	Nursing Intervention		
	Preprocedure	During Procedure	Postprocedure
Laryngoscopy or bronchoscopy	Explain the procedure, and clarify the client's concerns. Explain that a local spray or gargle will be given or that medications will be injected through a needle in the vein; that the client will rest the teeth against a small plastic mouthpiece; and that the procedure is painless but some pressure may be felt. Explain that the test will take about 30–60 minutes. Assess vital signs, sputum, and character of respirations for baseline data. Remove dentures, necklaces, ear rings, hairpins, and combs. Ensure good oral hygiene.	Assist the physician as required, for example, to hold the head piece or to move the client's head. Monitor the client's pulse and respirations. Support the client using touch and verbal communication.	1. Monitor vital signs q30min or as needed during the recovery period, and compare results to baseline data. 2. Withhold fluids until the gag reflex is restored and the client is conscious. 3. Position the client as ordered or indicated. Place the unconscious client in the lateral position so that secretions are not aspirated. 4. Inspect the client's sputum for blood caused by tissue damage. 5. Observe the client for signs of dyspnea, stridor, and shortness of breath, which may result from laryngeal edema or laryngospasm.

(*continued*)

G. Nursing Interventions for Endoscopic Examinations (*Continued*)

Examination	Nursing Intervention		
	Preprocedure	During Procedure	Postprocedure
Laryngoscopy or bronchoscopy (cont.)	Ensure that client is NPO for 6–8 hours beforehand. Confirm that the client is not allergic to any medications that will be given. Administer analgesic, sedative, antianxiety agent, and medication to dry secretions, if ordered.		6. Provide ice chips and warm saline gargles or throat lozenges, and administer ordered analgesics as required for throat discomfort. 7. Advise the client to contact the physician should difficulty with breathing, blood in sputum, fever, or pain occur.
Esophagoscopy, gastroscopy, and duodenoscopy	As above for bronchoscopy, with the exception of assessing sputum. Explain that the client may feel pressure in the stomach as the tube is moved about and feel fullness or bloating, like that after eating a large meal.	As above for bronchoscopy. Administer oral simethicone (Mylicon) before test if ordered; it decreases air bubbles in the stomach. If atropine is given intravenously to reduce gastrointestinal spasm, carefully monitor the client's pulse rate. Atropine increases the heart rate.	1. Follow steps 1–3 and 6, as for bronchoscopy. 2. Inspect vomitus for blood, and test it for occult blood if agency practice indicates. 3. Advise the client to contact the physician if client experiences persistent difficulty swallowing, pain, fever, blood in vomitus, or black stools.

Cystoscopy	Assess vital signs, frequency of urination, dysuria, and amount and consistency of urine for baseline data. Administer enema, if ordered. A clear bowel is necessary if x-ray studies are planned. If a general anesthetic is being given, ensure that client is NPO for 6–8 hours beforehand. For the client having a local anesthetic, provide appropriate fluid intake, if ordered, to ensure an adequate flow of urine for the collection of specimens. Administer sedative and medication to dry secretions, if ordered.	Support the client emotionally. Monitor vital signs. Label appropriately any specimens taken. Assist the primary care provider as requested.	1. Monitor vital signs, urination, and urine, and compare with baseline data. 2. Position the unconscious client appropriately (as for bronchoscopy). 3. Inspect the client's urine for blood; report bright red bleeding. 4. Report inability to urinate by 8 hours. 5. Encourage increased fluid intake to decrease irritation of urinary tissue. 6. If dyes were used in the procedure, warn the client that the urine may be an unusual color. 7. Administer analgesics, as ordered. 8. Advise the client to report persistent difficulty passing urine, bright blood in urine, pain, or fever.

(*continued*)

G. Nursing Interventions for Endoscopic Examinations (*Continued*)

Examination	Nursing Intervention		
	Preprocedure	During Procedure	Postprocedure
Anoscopy, proctoscopy, sigmoidoscopy, and colonoscopy	Assess vital signs and consistency of feces for baseline data. Ensure appropriate preexamination diet and fluid intake. Administer enemas until returns are clear, or suppository as ordered, the morning of the examination. Ensure that the client voids before the examination. The pressure during the procedure may injure a full bladder. Administer sedative beforehand, if ordered. Just before the endoscope is inserted, explain that the client may experience (a) sensation of having to move bowels (due to the pressure of the instrument) and (b) abdominal cramping when distending bowel with air.	Support the client physically in the genupectoral position, as needed. Monitor pulse and respiratory rates. Label appropriately any specimens taken. Support the client emotionally. Acknowledge feelings the client experiences (e.g., cramps) and ensure the client that they are not unusual.	1. Monitor vital signs and compare with baseline data. 2. Inspect the next few bowel move ments for blood. 3. Allow the client to rest. This proce dure may be physically and emotionally tiring. 4. Provide fluids and food.

H. Studies of the Gastrointestinal Tract

Name	Description	Nursing Intervention	
		Preprocedure	Postprocedure
Barium swallow	The client swallows barium, and the pharynx and esophagus are outlined on x-ray film.	Procedure lasts 30 minutes. Client is given a chalky substance (liquid barium) to drink.	Encourage fluids and activity to prevent constipation. Observe stool for whitish color indicating client has passed barium in stool. Notify primary care provider if barium does not pass in 2–3 days (a laxative may be required).
Upper gastrointestinal (UGI) series	The client swallows barium, and x-ray films are taken of its course through the esophagus, stomach, and duodenum.	Client must fast 4–6 hours before the examination. The client is given a chalky substance (liquid barium) to drink. Procedure lasts from 30 minutes to 1 hour. Client may experience a feeling of fullness. Client may need to assume several positions on the x-ray table.	Encourage fluids and activity to prevent constipation. Observe stool for whitish color, indicating client has passed barium in stool. Client may require a laxative or enema if client is constipated or does not pass barium in 2–3 days.

(*continued*)

H. Studies of the Gastrointestinal Tract (*Continued*)

Name	Description	Nursing Intervention	
		Preprocedure	Postprocedure
Lower gastrointestinal (LGI) series (barium enema)	A barium enema is given, and x-ray films are taken of the large intestine.	A laxative may be given the night before the test. Food is restricted after midnight before the test. Enemas or suppositories are given on the morning of the test to clean the bowel. The barium enema creates a feeling of fullness, and the client will feel the urge to defecate. Test usually lasts 30–45 minutes. There may be some cramping. Special tubes with balloons are often used to help the client retain the barium. The client is asked to assume various positions (e.g., left lateral, then right lateral) Client will probably pass the barium at the x-ray department.	Provide a rest period afterward; the procedure is fatiguing. Encourage fluids to prevent constipation. Observe stool for passage of barium, and assess regularity of bowel move ments. Notify primary care provider if barium does not pass in 2–3 days. An enema may be required if client does not pass all the barium.

I. Studies of the Gallbladder and Bile Ducts

Name	Description	Nursing Intervention	
		Preprocedure	Postprocedure
Cholecystography (oral cholecystography)	X-ray films are taken of the gallbladder after a contrast dye has been given orally.	A fat-free supper is given the evening before. Check for allergy to the contrast dye, which contains iodine. A laxative may be given the evening before, or an enema the morning of the test. Six or more contrast pills (e.g., Telepaque) are given in 5-minute intervals the evening before the test, each with 4–6 ounces of water. The client fasts from midnight the evening before but may drink water. Explain that (a) a fatty drink may be given during the test, (b) no discomfort is usually felt, and (c) the procedure lasts about 30–45 minutes.	Provide a rest period. Have client resume a regular diet. Provide a snack if the client is hungry. Assess allergy to the contrast dye.

(*continued*)

I. Studies of the Gallbladder and Bile Ducts (*Continued*)

Name	Description	Nursing Intervention	
		Preprocedure	Postprocedure
Intravenous cholangiography	X-ray films are taken of the bile ducts after dye has been administered intravenously.	The client fasts from midnight the evening before the test but may drink water. The bowel is cleaned with a laxative the evening before or with an enema the morning of the test. Check for allergy to iodine contained in the dye. Explain that iodine dye is given intravenously in the x-ray department. A test for allergy is given in the arm before the test.	Assess for allergy to the dye. Observe intravenous site for bleeding, tenderness.

Percutaneous transhepatic cholangiography	A needle is inserted through the abdominal wall into the biliary radicle, and a contrast agent is injected. Test distinguishes obstructive from nonobstructive jaundice.	Complete study lasts 3–4 hours. See preparation for intravenous cholangiography. Explain that procedure lasts approximately 30 minutes.	Monitor vital signs q15min for 1 hour, q30min for 4 hours, and then q4h until client is stable. Encourage bed rest. Position client on right side to place pressure on the puncture site to prevent bleeding.
Postoperative cholangiography	Dye is injected through the T-tube; x-ray films are taken and fluoroscopy is done to determine whether the common bile duct is unobstructed.	See preparation for intravenous cholangiography.	Monitor puncture site for bleeding. If T-tube is in place, clamp or attach to drainage as ordered. If T-tube is removed, apply sterile dressing.

J. Radiographic Studies: Intravenous Pyelography, Angiography, Myelography

Name	Description	Nursing Intervention	
		Preprocedure	Postprocedure
Intravenous pyelography or urography (IVP, IVU)	An intravenous injection of radiopaque material is given to examine the kidneys and ureters.	A strong laxative (e.g., castor oil) is given the afternoon before the test to clear the bowel of fecal material, which can obstruct the view of the urinary structures. The client fasts from midnight prior to the test. Check for allergy to iodine. Explain that (a) an intravenous injection will be administered in the x-ray department and (b) the procedure lasts about 1 hour.	Encourage fluid intake. The client resumes a regular diet. Provide for rest; the laxative and fasting can cause weakness. Observe for reactions to the radiopaque dye.

Angiography, for example, cerebral angiography (vascular system of the brain), coronary arteriography (coronary arteries), renal angiography (vascular system of the kidneys), pulmonary angiography (vascular system of the lungs)	A radiopaque material is injected into an artery or vein to examine portions of the vascular system.	For some of these procedures, a catheter may be inserted into an artery or vein prior to the injection of radiopaque material. Before some procedures, the client is given a sedative. The client fasts from midnight prior to the test. A strong laxative may be given the evening before certain tests (e.g., renal arteriography). Client is tested for allergy to iodine. The time needed for these procedures varies. Some may take up to 3 hours.	Bed rest is generally maintained for up to 12 hours. Monitor the client's radial pulse, respirations, and blood pressure q15–30min until they stabilize. Monitor peripheral pulses distal to the injection site. Observe the injection site for bleeding and swelling. Apply cold pack to prevent swelling. Determine any discomfort experienced by the client.

(*continued*)

J. Radiographic Studies: Intravenous Pyelography, Angiography, Myelography (*Continued*)

Name	Description	Nursing Intervention	
		Preprocedure	Postprocedure
Myelography	A contrast material is injected into the subarachnoid space, and x-ray films are taken of the spinal cord, nerve roots, and vertebrae.	Fasting may be required from midnight prior to the test. The client may be given a sedative before the procedure. Explain that (a) a radiopaque oil dye is injected via a lumbar puncture in the x-ray department; (b) the client will assume various positions (e.g., lateral for a lumbar puncture, then prone, and then tilted on x-ray table equipped with shoulder and foot supports); and (c) client may feel some pain when the oil is removed. The pain is due to irritation of the nerve roots. The procedure may last approximately 2 hours.	The client is generally positioned flat in bed for 24 hours to minimize headache and/or nausea; however, client may be positioned with the head elevated above the level of the spine if the dye has not been completely removed. This prevents the dye from moving to the head and causing an inflammation of the meninges (meningitis). Monitor vital signs and neurologic status (e.g., complaints of numb ness, pain, or tingling in the extremities; muscle weakness). Monitor urinary output.

K. Key Information About Vitamins

	RDA for Healthy Adults Ages 19–50	Major Dietary Sources	Major Functions	Signs of Severe, Prolonged Deficiency	Signs of Extreme Excess
Fat-Soluble Vitamins					
A (retinol)	Females: 700 RE; Males: 900 RE	Fat-containing and fortified dairy products; liver; provitamin carotene in orange and deep green fruits and vegetables	Vision growth; bone development; epithelial tissue formation; cellular differentiation	Night blindness; keratinization of epithelial tissues, including the cornea of the eye (xerophthalmia), causing permanent blind ness; dry, scaling skin; increased susceptibility to infection	Preformed vitamin A: damage to liver and bone; dry skin; headache; irritability; vomiting; hair loss; blurred vision Carotenoids: yellowed skin
D (calciferol)	15μg	Fortified and full-fat dairy products, fish liver oils, egg yolk (diet often not as important as sunlight exposure)	Promotes absorption and use of calcium and phosphorus	Rickets (bone deformities) in children; osteomalacia (bone softening) in adults	Calcium deposition in tissues leading to cerebral, cardiovascular, and kidney damage

(*continued*)

K. Key Information About Vitamins (*Continued*)

	RDA for Healthy Adults Ages 19–50	Major Dietary Sources	Major Functions	Signs of Severe, Prolonged Deficiency	Signs of Extreme Excess
E (tocopherol)	15 mg	Vegetable oils and their products; nuts, seeds	Antioxidant to prevent cell membrane damage	Possible anemia and neurologic effects	Generally nontoxic; may worsen clotting defect in vitamin K deficiency
K	Females: 90 µg Males: 120 µg	Green vegetables; green tea	Aids in formation of certain proteins, especially those for blood clotting	Defective blood coagulation causing severe bleeding on injury	Liver damage and anemia from high doses of the synthetic form (menadione)
Water-Soluble Vitamins					
Thiamin (B_1)	Females: 1.1 mg Males: 1.2 mg	Brewer's yeast, pork, legumes, peanuts, enriched or whole-grain products	Coenzyme used in energy metabolism	Dementia; paralysis; neuropathy; edema; beriberi	Generally nontoxic

Riboflavin (B_2)	Females: 1.1 mg Males: 1.3 mg	Beef liver, dairy products, meats, eggs, enriched grain products	Coenzyme used in energy metabolism	Skin lesions	Generally nontoxic
Niacin	Females: 14 niacin equivalents Males: 16 niacin equivalents	Nuts, meats; provitamin tryptophan in most proteins	Coenzyme used in energy metabolism	Pellagra (multiple vitamin deficiencies, including niacin)	Flushing of face, neck, hands; potential liver damage
B_6 (pyridoxine)	1.3 mg	Yeast, wheat germ, liver, high-protein foods in general	Coenzyme used in amino acid metabolism	Nervous, skin, and muscular disorders; anemia	Ataxia, neuropathy
Folic acid (folate)	400 µg	Liver, beans, green vegetables, oranges, nuts, grain products	Coenzyme used in DNA and RNA metabolism; single carbon utilization	Megaloblastic anemia (large, immature red blood cells); gastrointestinal disturbances	Generally nontoxic
B_{12} (cobalamin)	2.4 µg	Animal products	Coenzyme used in DNA and RNA metabolism; single carbon utilization	Megaloblastic anemia; pernicious anemia when due to inadequate intrinsic factor; nervous system damage	Thought to be nontoxic

(*continued*)

K. Key Information About Vitamins (*Continued*)

	RDA for Healthy Adults Ages 19–50	Major Dietary Sources	Major Functions	Signs of Severe, Prolonged Deficiency	Signs of Extreme Excess
Pantothenic acid	5 mg	Animal products and whole grains; widely distributed in foods	Coenzyme used in energy metabolism	None	Generally nontoxic; occasionally causes diarrhea
Biotin	30 µg	Widely distributed in foods	Coenzyme used in energy metabolism	Scaly dermatitis	Thought to be nontoxic
C (ascorbic acid)	90 mg	Fruits and vegetables, especially broccoli, cabbage, cantaloupe, cauliflower, citrus fruits, green pepper, kiwi fruit, strawberries	Functions in synthesis of collagen; is an antioxidant; aids in detoxification; improves iron absorption; still under intense study	Scurvy; petechiae (minute hemorrhages around hair follicles); weakness; delayed wound healing; impaired immune response	Gastrointestinal upset; interferes with certain lab tests

From: *DRI: Dietary Reference Intakes: The Essential Guide to Nutrient Requirements*. (2006). Washington, DC: National Academies Press. Retrieved from http://fnic.nal.usda.gov/interactiveDRI/

L. Key Information About Minerals

Major Mineral	RDA for Healthy Adults Ages 19–50	Major Dietary Sources	Major Functions	Signs of Severe, Prolonged Deficiency	Signs of Extreme Excess
Calcium	1000 mg	Milk, cheese, dark green vegetables, legumes	Bone and tooth formation; blood clotting; nerve transmission	Stunted growth; perhaps less bone mass; hypertension	Depressed absorption of some other minerals; perhaps kidney damage
Chloride	2.3 gm	Same as for sodium	Plays a role in acid–base balance; formation of gastric juice	Muscle cramps; reduced appetite; poor growth	High blood pressure in genetically predisposed individuals
Magnesium	Females: 320 mg Males: 420 mg	Whole grains, green leafy vegetables	Component of enzymes	Neurologic disturbances	Neurologic disturbances
Phosphorus	700 mg	Milk, cheese, meat, poultry, whole grains	Bone and tooth formation; acid-base balance; component of coenzymes	Weakness; demineralization of bone	Depressed absorption of some minerals

(*Continued*)

L. Key Information About Minerals(*Continued*)

Major Mineral	RDA for Healthy Adults Ages 19–50	Major Dietary Sources	Major Functions	Signs of Severe, Prolonged Deficiency	Signs of Extreme Excess
Potassium	4.7 gm	Meats, milk, many fruits and vegetables, whole grains	Body water balance; nerve function	Muscular weakness; paralysis	Muscular weakness; cardiac arrest
Sodium	1.5 gm	Salt, soy sauce, cured meats, pickles, canned soups, processed cheese	Body water balance; nerve function	Muscle cramps; reduced appetite	High blood pressure in genetically predisposed individuals
Sulfur	(Provided by sulfur amino acids)*	Sulfur amino acids in dietary proteins	Component of cartilage, tendons, and proteins	Related to protein deficiency	Excess sulfur-containing amino acid intake leads to poor growth; liver damage

*No formal recommendation.

M. Key Information about Trace Minerals

Trace Mineral	RDA for Healthy Adults Ages 19–50	Major Dietary Sources	Major Functions	Signs of Severe, Prolonged Deficiency	Signs of Extreme Excess
Chromium	Females: 25 µg† Males: 35 µg	Brewer's yeast, liver, seafood, meat, potatoes	Involved in glucose and energy metabolism	Impaired glucose metabolism	Lung and kidney damage (occupational exposures only)
Cobalt	(Required as vitamin B_{12})*	Animal products	Component of vitamin B_{12}	Not reported except as vitamin B_{12} deficiency	Polycythemia
Copper	900 µg†	Seafood, nuts, legumes, organ meats	Component of enzymes	Anemia; bone and cardiovascular changes	Nausea; liver damage
Fluoride	Females: 3 mg Males: 4 mg†	Drinking water, tea, seafood	Maintenance of tooth (and maybe bone) structure	Higher frequency of tooth decay	Acute: gastrointestinal distress Chronic: mottling of teeth; skeletal deformation

(*Continued*)

M. Key Information about Trace Minerals (*Continued*)

Trace Mineral	RDA for Healthy Adults Ages 19–50	Major Dietary Sources	Major Functions	Signs of Severe, Prolonged Deficiency	Signs of Extreme Excess
Iodine	150 µg	Fish and shellfish, dairy products, iodized salt, some breads	Component of thyroid hormones	Goiter (enlarged thyroid); mental retardation	Goiter
Iron	Females: 8 mg Males: 8 mg	Meats, eggs, beans, whole grains, green leafy vegetables	Components of hemoglobin, myoglobin, and enzymes	Iron-deficiency anemia; weakness; impaired immune function	Acute: shock; death Chronic: liver damage; cardiac failure
Manganese	Females: 1.8 mg Males: 2.3 mg	Nuts, whole grains, vegetables and fruits, tea	Component of enzymes	Abnormal bone and cartilage; sterility	Central nervous system damage (occupational exposures)
Molybdenum	45 µg†	Beans, cereals, dark green, leafy vegetables	Component of enzymes	Disorder in nitrogen excretion; mental changes	Inhibition of enzymes; gout-like syndrome

Selenium	55 µg	Seafood, meats, whole grains, Brazil nuts	Component of enzymes; functions in close association with vitamin E	Muscle pain; maybe heart muscle deterioration	Unknown
Zinc	Females: 8 mg Males: 11 mg	Meats, seafood, whole grains	Component of enzymes	Growth failure; scaly dermatitis; reproductive failure; impaired immune function	Acute: nausea; vomiting; diarrhea Chronic: adversely affects copper metabolism and immune function; anemia

From: DRI: *Dietary Reference Intakes: The Essential Guide to Nutrient Requirements.* (2006). Washington, DC: National Academies Press. Retrieved from http://fnic.nal.usda.gov/interactiveDRI/

*No formal recommendation.

†Estimated safe and adequate daily dietary intake.

GLOSSARY

abduction movement of a body part away from the midline of the body

abrasion scraping away of the surface of a structure, such as the skin or teeth

abscess a localized collection of pus and disintegrating body cells

absorption (of drug) the process by which a drug passes into the bloodstream

acidosis (acidemia) a condition that occurs with increases in blood carbonic acid or with decreases in blood bicarbonate; arterial blood pH below 7.35

acromion (acromial process) the lateral projection of the scapula extending over the shoulder joint

activities of daily living (ADLs) the tasks of daily life, such as eating, bathing, and dressing

acute sharp or severe; describing a severe condition with a sudden onset and short course (as opposed to chronic)

adduction movement of a body part toward the midline of the body

adipose fat; of a fatty nature

adventitious breath sounds abnormal breath sounds

aldosterone a hormone produced by the adrenal cortex that regulates the level of sodium in the body

alkalosis (alkalemia) a condition that occurs with increases in blood bicarbonate or decreases in blood carbonic acid; arterial blood pH above 7.45

alopecia abnormal loss of hair

ampule a small, sealed glass flask, usually designed to hold a single dose of medication

analgesic a medication used to decrease pain

anaphylaxis (anaphylactic shock, anaphylactic reaction) a severe allergic reaction

anemia a condition in which the blood is deficient in red blood cells or hemoglobin

anesthesia loss of sensation or feeling; induced loss of the sense of pain

aneurysm dilation of the wall of an artery or vein

angiography a diagnostic procedure allowing x-ray visualization of the vascular system after injection of a radiopaque dye
anorexia lack of appetite
anoxia systemic absence or reduction of oxygen in the body tissues below physiological levels
anterior or at the front of
antibiotic a substance that has the capacity to inhibit the growth of or kill microorganisms
antibody (immunoglobulin) a protective substance produced in the body to counteract antigens
antidiuretic hormone (ADH) a hormone that is stored and released by the posterior pituitary gland and that controls water reabsorption from the kidney tubules; also referred to as *vasopressin*
antigen a substance capable of inducing the formation of antibodies
antipyretic a substance that is effective in reducing fever
antiseptic an agent that inhibits the growth of some microorganisms
anuria the failure of the kidneys to produce urine, resulting in total lack of urination or output of less than 100 mL per day in an adult
aphasia the inability to communicate by speech, signs, or writing, resulting from an injury or disease
apical pulse the central pulse, located at the apex of the heart
apical-radial pulse simultaneous measurement of the apical beat and the radial pulse
apnea cessation of breathing
approximate to bring close together (referring to wound or incision edges)
arrhythmia an irregular cardiac rhythm
arteriosclerosis a condition in which the walls of the arteries become hardened, thickened, and less compliant
ascites the accumulation of fluid in the abdominal cavity
asepsis freedom from infection or infectious material
asphyxia a condition resulting from a lack of oxygen
aspirate to remove gases or fluids from a cavity by using suction
astringent an agent that causes contraction or shrinkage of tissue; usually applied topically
ataxia failure of muscle coordination
atelectasis collapse of lung tissue
atony lack of normal muscle tone
atrophy a wasting away or decrease in size of a cell, tissue, body organ, or muscle
auscultation the practice of examining the body by listening to body sounds
axilla the armpit (plural: axillae)
axillary line an imaginary line extending vertically from the anterior fold of the axilla
bacteriuria bacteria in the urine
barium a metallic element commonly used in solution as a contrast medium for x-ray filming of the gastrointestinal tract

barium enema x-ray filming of the large intestine using a contrast medium; also called a *lower gastrointestinal series*

barium swallow x-ray filming of the esophagus, stomach, and duodenum; also referred to as an *upper gastrointestinal series*

barrel chest a chest shape in which the ratio of the anteroposterior diameter to the lateral diameter is 1 to 1

basal metabolic rate (BMR) the rate of energy utilization in the body required to maintain body functions at rest

bilateral affecting two sides

bilirubin orange or yellow pigment in the bile

binder a type of bandage applied to large body areas, such as the abdomen or chest

biopsy the removal and examination of tissue from the living body

bleb (wheal) a small, smooth, slightly raised area on the skin, usually filled with fluid

brachial pulse a pulse located on the inner side of the biceps muscle just below the axilla; usually palpated medially in the antecubital space

bradycardia an abnormally slow heart rate, below 60 beats per minute in an adult

bronchial sounds normal loud, harsh, hollow blowing sounds heard by auscultation over the trachea and major bronchi

bronchodilator an agent that dilates the bronchi of the lungs

bronchopneumonia an infection that originates in the bronchi and involves patches of lung tissue

bronchoscope a lighted instrument used to visualize the bronchi of the lungs

bronchovesicular sounds combination of bronchial and vesicular sounds heard by auscultation over parts of the chest where a bronchus is near lung tissue

bruxism grinding of the teeth during sleep

buccal pertaining to the cheek

buffer an agent or system that tends to maintain constancy of or that prevents changes in the chemical concentration of a substance

bulimia an uncontrollable compulsion to consume enormous amounts of food and then expel the food by self-induced vomiting or by taking laxatives

calculus a stone composed of minerals that is formed in the body, for example, a renal calculus formed in the kidney

cannula a tube with a lumen (channel), which is inserted into a cavity or duct and is often fitted with a trocar during insertion

canthus the angle formed by the upper and lower eyelids; each eye has an inner and an outer canthus

cardiac arrest the cessation of heart function

cardiac output the amount of blood ejected from the heart per minute by ventricular contraction; it is the stroke volume times the heart rate per minute

cardiopulmonary resuscitation (CPR) artificial stimulation of the heart and lungs; also referred to as *basic life support (BLS)*

caries decay of a tooth or bone
carina the ridge or junction where the main bronchi meet the trachea
carminative an agent that prevents the formation of gas in the colon
carotid arteries major arteries lying on either side of the trachea and larynx
cataract opacity of the lens of the eye or its capsule
cathartic (laxative) a drug that induces evacuation of feces from the large intestine
catheter a tube of plastic, rubber, metal, or other material used to remove or inject fluids into a cavity, such as the bladder
caudal anesthetic an anesthetic injected into the caudal canal, below the spinal cord
cellulitis inflammation of cellular tissue
centigrade (Celsius) a thermometer scale used to measure heat; the freezing point of water is 0°C, and the boiling point is 100°C
central venous pressure (CVP) a measurement of the pressure of the blood, in millimeters of water, within the vena cava or the right atrium of the heart
cephalocaudal proceeding in the direction from head to toe
cerebrospinal fluid fluid contained within the four ventricles of the brain, the subarachnoid space, and the central canal of the spinal cord
cerumen waxlike material found in the external auditory canal
chancre a papular lesion (sore) occurring at the primary site of infection in some diseases; the primary sore of syphilis
Cheyne-Stokes respirations rhythmic waxing and waning of respirations from very deep breathing to very shallow breathing with periods of temporary apnea; often associated with cardiac failure, increased intracranial pressure, or brain damage
chill shivering and shaking of the body with involuntary contractions of the voluntary muscles
cholangiogram an x-ray film of the biliary tract taken after the injection of a dye
cholecystogram an x-ray film of the gallbladder after the ingestion of a contrast dye; also called *oral cholecystography*
cholesterol a lipid that does not contain fatty acid but possesses many of the chemical and physical properties of other lipids
chronic persisting over a long time
chyme semifluid material produced by gastric digestion of food in the stomach; it is found in the small and large intestines
cicatrix scar
cilia hairlike projections from cells, for example, cells of the mucous membrane of the respiratory tract
circulatory overload a state of increased blood volume
circumduction movement of the distal part of a bone in a circle, with the proximal end remaining fixed
clean technique a technique that maintains an area or articles free from infectious agents

closed wound a wound in which there is no break in the skin

clubbing (of nails) an elevation of the proximal aspect of the nail and softening of the nail bed

coagulate to clot

cochlea a tubular structure in the inner ear that contains the organ for hearing

colic paroxysmal intestinal cramplike pain

collagen a protein found in connective tissue; a whitish protein substance that adds tensile strength to a wound

colonoscope a lighted instrument used to visualize the interior of the colon

colostomy an artificial abdominal opening into the colon (large bowel)

comatose a state of unconsciousness in which the person shows no response to maximum painful stimuli, absence of reflexes, and absence of muscle tone in the extremities

commode a portable chairlike structure used as a toilet

communicable disease (infectious disease) a disease that can spread from one person to another

compliance (vascular) distensibility or the ability to contract and expand

congenital existing at, and often before, birth

conjunctiva the delicate membrane that covers the eyeball and lines the eyelids

conjunctivitis inflammation of the conjunctiva

consciousness a person's normal state of awareness of the environment, self, and others

consensual reaction (of the eyes) a reaction in which one pupil constricts quickly in response to a bright light and the other pupil constricts also, but more slowly

constipation passage of small, dry, hard stool or passage of no stool for an abnormally long time

contaminated possessing disease-producing microorganisms

contracture permanent shortening of a muscle and subsequent shortening of tendons and ligaments

contusion a closed wound that occurs as a result of a blow from a blunt instrument; a bruise

core temperature temperature of the deep structures of the body

cornea the transparent covering of the anterior eye that connects with the sclera

costal angle the angle formed between the ribs and the sternum

costal (thoracic) breathing breathing using chiefly the intercostal muscles

costovertebral angle the angle formed by a rib and the spine

counterirritant an agent that produces an irritation with the intent of relieving some other problem

crackles (rales) rattling or bubbling breath sounds generally heard on inspiration

creatinine a nitrogenous waste that is excreted in the urine

Credé's maneuver manual exertion of pressure on the bladder to force urine out

crepitus (crepitation) skeletal: a grating sound caused by bone fragments rubbing together; respiratory: a dry, crackling sound like that of crumpled cellophane, produced by air in the subcutaneous tissue or by air moving through fluid in the alveoli of the lungs

culture in microbiology, the cultivation of microorganisms or cells in a special growth medium

cyanosis bluish discoloration of the skin, nail beds, and mucous membranes, due to reduced oxygen in the blood

cyst an enclosed cavity or sac lined by epithelium and containing liquid or semisolid material

cystitis inflammation of the urinary bladder

cystoscope a lighted instrument used to visualize the interior of the urinary bladder

cystoscopy visual examination of the urinary bladder with a cystoscope

cytology the study of the origin, structure, function, and pathology of cells

debride to remove foreign and dying tissue from a wound so that healthy tissue is exposed

defecation expulsion of feces from the rectum and anus

dehiscence a splitting open or rupture

dehydration insufficient fluid in the body

dementia decline in memory and other cognitive abilities

dependent edema edema that collects in the lower parts of the body, where hydrostatic pressure is greatest

dermatitis inflammation of the skin

dermatologic preparation a medication applied to the skin

dermis (corium) true skin, containing blood vessels, nerves, hair follicles, and glands

detrusor muscle the three layers of smooth muscle that make up the urinary bladder

dextrose a sugar; also called *glucose*

diagnosis a statement or conclusion concerning the nature of some phenomenon

diaphoresis profuse sweating

diaphragmatic (abdominal) breathing breathing that chiefly involves movement of the diaphragm and the abdomen

diarrhea defecation of liquid feces and increased frequency of defecation

diastole the period when the ventricles of the heart are relaxed

diastolic pressure the pressure of the blood against the arterial walls when the ventricles of the heart are at rest

digital performed with the finger

disorientation a state of mental confusion; loss of bearings, time, and place

distal farthest from the point of reference
diuresis see *polyuria*
diuretic an agent that increases the production of urine
dorsal of, toward, or at the back
dorsal flexion movement of the ankle so that the toes point up
dorsalis pedis pulse a pulse located on the instep of the foot
dorsal recumbent position a back-lying position with the head and shoulders slightly elevated
drainage a discharge from a wound or cavity
drug interaction the beneficial or harmful interaction of one drug with another drug
drug tolerance a condition in which successive increases in the dosage of a drug are required to maintain a given therapeutic effect
drug toxicity the quality of a drug that exerts a deleterious effect on an organism or tissue
dullness (in percussion) decreased resonance or percussion sound that occurs over dense tissue or large amounts of fluid
dysmenorrhea painful menstruation
dyspepsia indigestion
dysphagia difficulty or inability to swallow
dysphasia difficulty speaking
dysphoria a feeling of disquiet, restlessness, anxiety, depression
dyspnea difficult and labored breathing in which the client has a persistent unsatisfied need for air
dysrhythmia an irregular cardiac rhythm
dysuria painful or difficult urination
ecchymosis a blotchy area of discoloration of the skin; a bruise
edema excess interstitial fluid
electrocardiogram (ECG, EKG) a graph of the electric activity of the heart
electroencephalogram (EEG) a graph of the electric activity of the brain
electrolyte ionized salts found in cells, tissue fluids, and blood
embolus a blood clot (or a substance, such as air) that has moved from its place of origin and is obstructing the circulation in a blood vessel (plural: emboli)
emollient an agent that soothes and softens skin or mucous membrane; often an oily substance
emphysema a chronic obstructive lung disorder in which the terminal bronchioles become distended and plugged with mucus
emulsion a preparation in which one liquid is distributed throughout another
endogenous developing from within
endoscope a lighted instrument used to visualize the interior of a hollow organ
endothelium the layer of endothelial cells lining the blood vessels, cavities of the heart, and serous cavities
endotracheal tube a tube inserted into the trachea

enema a solution injected into the rectum and the sigmoid colon
enteric referring to the small intestines
enteric coated surrounded with a special coating used for tablets and capsules that prevents release of the drug until it is in the intestines
enteric feeding a feeding administered directly into the small intestine through a tube
enterostomal therapist a person who specializes in ostomy care
enzyme a biologic catalyst that induces chemical reactions
epidemic the occurrence of a disease in many people at the same time or in rapid succession in an area
epidermis the outermost, nonvascular layer of skin
epistaxis nosebleed
eructation ejection of gas from the stomach (belching)
erythema redness that is associated with a variety of rashes
erythrocyte red blood cell
eschar a slough of dried plasma proteins and dead cells; often produced by a burn, corrosive application, or gangrene
esophagoscopy visual examination of the interior of the esophagus with a lighted instrument
etiology cause
eupnea normal respiration that is quiet, rhythmic, and effortless
evisceration removal of or spilling out of the internal organs
exanthema skin rash
excise to cut off or out
excoriation abrasion of the superficial layers of the skin
excretion elimination of waste products from the body
exogenous developing from without
expectorate to cough and spit up mucus or other materials
expiratory reserve volume the maximum amount of air exhaled after a normal exhalation
extension increasing the angle of a joint (between two bones); the act of straightening
external cardiac massage rhythmic massage of the heart muscle over the sternum
extracellular outside the cells
extracellular fluid (ECF) fluid found outside the body cells
extravasation the escape of blood from a vessel into body tissues
exudate material, such as fluid and cells, that has escaped from blood vessels and is deposited in tissues or on tissue surfaces during the inflammatory process
febrile pertaining to a fever; feverish
fecal impaction a mass of hardened feces in the rectum
fecal incontinence inability to control the passage of feces through the anus
feces (stool) body wastes and undigested food eliminated from the rectum
femoral pulse the pulse found in the groin at the midpoint of the inguinal ligament

fever elevated body temperature

fibrillation involuntary contractions of a muscle; cardiac arrhythmia characterized by extremely rapid, irregular, and ineffective contractions of the atria or ventricles

first intention healing primary healing of a wound, which occurs when the tissue surfaces have been approximated

fistula an abnormal communication or passage, usually between two organs or between an organ and the body surface

flaccid weak or lax

flaccid paralysis impaired muscle function with loss of muscle tone

flail chest a condition of the chest wall caused by two or more rib fractures resulting in paradoxical breathing

flatness (in percussion) absence of resonance; extreme dullness

flatulence the presence of excessive amounts of gas in the stomach or intestines

flatus gas or air normally present in the stomach or intestines

flexion decreasing the angle of a joint (between two bones); the act of bending

flow sheet a record used to chart the progress of specific or specialized data, such as vital signs, fluid balance, or routine medications

fluoroscope a device for examining internal structures using roentgen (x-) rays

flushing (of the skin) transient redness of the skin, often of the face and neck; it may be generalized or restricted to a particular area

footdrop plantar flexion of the foot with permanent contracture of the gastrocnemius (calf) muscle and tendon

forceps an instrument with two blades and a handle used to grasp sterile supplies and to compress or grasp tissues

foreskin a covering fold of skin over the glans of the penis; also called the *prepuce*

formulary a collection or list of prescriptions and formulas

Fowler's position a bed-sitting position with the head of the bed raised to 45 degrees

fracture a break in the continuity of bone

fremitus vibration perceptible on palpation

frenulum a fold of mucous membrane that attaches the tongue to the floor of the mouth; a fold on the lower surface of the glans penis that connects it with the prepuce

friction rub see *pleural rub*

gait the way a person walks

gastric pertaining to the stomach

gastrocolic reflex increased peristalsis of the colon after food has entered the stomach

gastroenteritis inflammation of the stomach and the intestines

gastroscopy visual examination of the stomach with a gastroscope

gastrostomy a surgical opening that leads through the abdomen directly into the stomach

gauge (of a needle) the diameter of the shaft of a needle
gavage administration of nourishment to the stomach through a nasogastric or orogastric tube; tube feeding
generic name a drug name not protected by trademark and usually describing the chemical structure of the drug
gingivitis inflammation of the gums
glans penis the cap-shaped, expansive structure at the end of the penis
glaucoma an eye disease characterized by an increase in intraocular pressure that produces changes in the optic disc and the field of vision
glomerular filtrate fluid formed in the nephron of the kidney that is similar to plasma in composition; the precursor of urine
glossitis inflammation of the tongue
glottis the vocal apparatus of the larynx
glucose a monosaccharide occurring in food
glycogen the chief carbohydrate stored in the body, particularly in the liver and muscles
glycosuria the presence of glucose in the urine; glucosuria
gonorrhea a sexually transmitted disease due to Neisseria gonorrhoeae infection
gout a condition characterized by excessive uric acid in the blood
granulation tissue young connective tissue with new capillaries formed in the wound-healing process
half-life (of drug) the time interval required for the body's elimination processes to reduce the concentration of the drug in the body by one half
halitosis bad breath
hallux valgus bunion or lateral deviation of the big toe
Heimlich maneuver subdiaphragmatic abdominal thrusts used to clear an obstructed airway
hemangioma a large, persistent, bright red or dark purple vascular area of the skin
hematemesis the vomiting of blood
hematocrit the percentage of red blood cell mass in proportion to whole blood
hematoma a collection of blood in a tissue, organ, or body space due to a break in the wall of a blood vessel
hematuria the presence of blood in the urine
hemiplegia the loss of movement on one side of the body
hemoglobin the red pigment in red blood cells that carries oxygen
hemoglobinuria the presence of hemoglobin in the urine
hemolysis rupture of red blood cells
hemopneumothorax a collection of blood and air or gas in the pleural cavity
hemoptysis the presence of blood in the sputum
hemorrhage bleeding; the escape of blood from the blood vessels
hemorrhoids distended veins in the anus and rectum

hemothorax a collection of blood in the pleural cavity
heparin a substance that prevents coagulation of blood
heparin lock an indwelling intravenous catheter attached to a sealed injection tip
hernia protrusion of an organ or tissue through an opening in the wall of the cavity that usually contains it
hesitancy (of urination) delay and difficulty initiating voiding
high Fowler's position a bed-sitting position in which the head of the bed is elevated 90 degrees
hirsutism abnormal hairiness, particularly in women
Homan's sign calf pain produced by dorsiflexion of the foot, an early sign of venous thrombosis
homeostasis tendency of the body to maintain a state of balance or equilibrium while continually changing
humidifier a device that adds water vapor to inspired air
hydration the addition of water to a substance or tissue
hydrocephalus a disease process resulting in excessive cerebrospinal fluid within the ventricles of the brain
hydrocortisone an adrenocorticosteroid produced by the adrenal glands or produced synthetically; also called *cortisol*
hyperalgesia extreme sensitivity to pain
hyperalimentation see *total parenteral nutrition*
hypercalcemia excessive calcium in the blood plasma
hypercalciuria excessive calcium in the urine
hypercarbia (hypercapnia) accumulation of carbon dioxide in the blood
hyperemia increased blood flow to an area
hyperextension further extension between two bones or stretching out of a joint
hyperglycemia an increased concentration of glucose in the blood
hyperhidrosis excessive perspiration
hyperkalemia excessive potassium in the blood
hyperlipidemia elevated concentration of lipids in the plasma
hypermagnesemia excessive magnesium in the blood plasma
hypernatremia an elevated level of sodium in the blood plasma
hyperplasia an abnormal increase in the number of normal cells in a tissue or an organ
hyperpnea an increase in the rate of breathing or an increase in depth of respirations
hyperpyrexia an extremely elevated body temperature
hyperreflexia an exaggeration of the reflexes
hyperresonance a sound that is lower-pitched than resonance; booming sound
hypersensitivity an exaggerated response of the body to a foreign substance
hypersomnia excessive sleep
hypertension an abnormally high blood pressure

hyperthermia an abnormally high body temperature, sometimes induced as a therapeutic measure
hypertonicity excessive muscle tone or activity
hypertonic solution a fluid possessing a greater concentration of solutes than plasma
hypertrophy an increase in size of a cell, tissue, or body organ, such as a muscle
hyperventilation an increase in the amount of air entering the lungs, characterized by deep, rapid breaths
hypervolemia an abnormal increase in the body's blood volume; circulatory overload
hypnotic (drug) a drug that induces sleep
hypoalbuminemia reduction in the level of albumin in the blood
hypocalcemia decreased calcium in the blood plasma
hypoglycemia a reduced amount of glucose in the blood
hypokalemia potassium deficit in the blood plasma
hypomagnesemia low magnesium in the blood plasma
hyponatremia an abnormally low amount of sodium in the blood plasma
hypoproteinemia decreased amount of protein in the blood plasma
hypostatic pneumonia an infection of lung tissue resulting from poor circulation or stagnation of secretions
hypotension an abnormally low blood pressure
hypothermia an abnormally low body temperature
hypotonicity decreased muscle tone
hypotonic solution a fluid possessing a lesser concentration of solutes than plasma
hypoventilation a reduction in the amount of air entering the lungs, characterized by shallow respirations
hypovolemia decreased blood volume
hypovolemic shock a state of shock due to a reduction in the volume of circulating blood
hypoxemia low partial pressure of oxygen or low saturation of oxyhemoglobin in the arterial blood
hypoxia oxygen deficiency
iatrogenic caused by the physician or medical therapy
ileal conduit method of diverting urinary flow into a piece of ileum
ileostomy an artificial abdominal opening into the ileum (small bowel)
immobility prescribed or unavoidable restriction of movement in any area of a person's life
immunity a specific resistance of the body to infection; it may be naturally endowed resistance or resistance developed after exposure to a disease agent
immunization the process of becoming immune or rendering someone immune
immunoglobulin a part of the body's plasma proteins; also called *immune bodies* or *antibodies*

impaction a condition of being firmly wedged or lodged; in reference to feces, a collection of hardened puttylike feces in the folds of the rectum

incentive spirometer (sustained maximal inspiration [SMI] device) a device that measures the flow of air through a mouthpiece as the client practices maximal depth of respiration

incision a cut or wound that is intentionally made, for example, during surgery

incompatibility (of drug) undesired chemical or physical reaction between a drug and an infusion solution, between two or more drugs, or between a drug and the container or tubing

incontinence inability to control the elimination of urine (enuresis) or feces (fecal incontinence)

incubation period the time between the entry of microorganisms into the body and the onset of symptoms of the infection

induration hardening

infarct a localized area of necrosis (dead cells) usually caused by obstructed arterial blood flow to the part

infection the disease process produced by microorganisms

infiltration the diffusion or deposition of substances into a tissue

inflammation local and nonspecific defensive tissue response to injury or destruction of cells

infusion the introduction of fluid into a vein or part of the body

inhalation (aerosol) therapy delivery of droplets of medication or moisture suspended in a gas, such as oxygen, by inhalation through the nose or mouth

insomnia inability to initiate or maintain a sufficient quality or quantity of sleep

inspection visual examination to detect features perceptible to the eye

instillation application of a medication into a body cavity or orifice

insulin a hormone secreted by the beta cells of the islets of Langerhans in the pancreas

integument the skin or covering of the body

intercostal between the ribs

intercostal retractions indrawing between the ribs with inspiration

internal rotation a turning toward the midline, such as rotation of the hip joint

interstitial between the cells of the body's tissues

interstitial fluid fluid surrounding the body cells

intestinal distention stretching and inflation of the intestines due to the presence of air or gas

intracellular within a cell or cells

intracellular fluid (cellular fluid, ICF) fluid found within the body cells

intractable pain pain that is resistant to cure or relief

intradermal (intracutaneous) within the skin

intramuscular within or inside muscle tissue

intraoperative period the time during surgery

intrapleural within the pleural cavity

intrathecal within or into the spinal canal
intravascular within a blood vessel
intravenous within a vein
intravenous cholangiogram an x-ray film of the bile ducts after a contrast dye has been administered intravenously
intravenous push (IVP, bolus) direct intravenous administration of a medication
intravenous pyelogram an x-ray film of the kidneys taken after intravenous injection of a radiopaque dye
intravenous pyelography (IVP) x-ray filming of the kidney and ureters after injection of a radiopaque material intravenously; also called *intravenous urography*
intravertebral (intraspinal) within the vertebrae
intubation insertion of a tube
inversion a turning inward
ion an atom with an electric charge
iron-deficiency anemia form of anemia caused by an inadequate supply of iron for synthesis of hemoglobin
irradiation exposure to penetrating rays, such as x-rays, gamma rays, infrared rays, or ultraviolet rays
irrigation (lavage) the washing of a body cavity or a wound
irritant a substance that stimulates unpleasant responses, that is, irritates
ischemia lack of blood supply to a body part
isolation practice that prevents the spread of infection and communicable diseases
isometric having the same measure or length
isotonic having the same tonicity as the body fluids; the term is used to compare solutions of the same strength or concentration
jaundice a yellowish tinge to the skin and mucous membrane caused by excess bilirubin in the blood
jejunum the portion of the small intestine that extends from the duodenum to the ileum
Kardex a portable card index file that organizes data about clients in a concise way and, often, contains nursing care plans
Kegel's exercises exercises for tightening pelvic floor or perineal muscles
ketosis a condition in which excessive ketones are accumulated in the body
Korotkoff's sounds a series of five sounds heard when auscultating blood pressure; these sounds are produced by blood within the artery with each ventricular contraction
kyphosis an exaggerated convexity in the thoracic region of the vertebral column, resulting in a stooped posture
labored breathing difficult or dyspneic breathing
lacerate to tear, rather than cut, a body tissue
lacrimal sac the opening connecting the tear ducts in the inner canthus of the eye to the nasolacrimal duct, which empties into the nasal cavity

lacrimation the secretion and discharge of tears
laryngeal stridor a harsh, crowing sound heard during expiration when a laryngeal obstruction is present
laryngoscopy visual examination of the larynx with a laryngoscope
laryngospasm spasmodic closure of the larynx
lateral to the side, away from the midline
lateral position a side-lying position
lavage an irrigation or washing of a body organ, such as the stomach
laxative a medication that stimulates bowel activity
lentigo senilis clusters of melanocytes that appear as brown "age" spots
lesion the traumatic or pathologic interruption of a tissue or the loss of function of a body part
lethargy drowsiness; a state in which a person sleeps much of the time when the person is not stimulated
leukocyte a white blood cell
leukocytosis an increase in the number of white blood cells
Levin tube a single-lumen nasogastric tube
ligament a broad, fibrous band that holds two or more bones together
liniment a topical liquid applied to the skin frequently to stimulate circulation or to relieve pain
lithotomy position a back-lying position in which the feet are supported in stirrups
lobar pneumonia an infectious disease of one or more lobes of the lung
lobe a well-defined portion of an organ, for example, of the lung or brain
lordosis an exaggerated concavity in the lumbar region of the vertebral column
lumbar puncture (LP, spinal tap) the insertion of a needle into the subarachnoid space at the lumbar region
lumen a channel within a tube, such as the channel of an artery in which blood flows
lung compliance expansibility of the lung
lung recoil the tendency of lungs to collapse away from the chest wall
lymphatic referring to lymph or lymph vessels
maceration the wasting away or softening of a solid as if by the action of soaking
malaise a general feeling of being unwell or indisposed
malignancy abnormal tissue with a tendency to grow and invade other tissues
malleolus a rounded prominence on the distal end of the tibia or fibula
malnutrition a disorder of nutrition; insufficient nourishment of the body cells
mammography x-ray study of breast tissues
mastectomy surgical removal of the breast

masticate to chew
meatus an opening, passage, or channel
medial toward the middle or midline
medical asepsis practices that limit the number, growth, and spread of microorganisms; clean technique
melanin the dark pigment of the skin
meniscus the crescent-shaped structure of the surface of a column of liquid; the crescent-shaped cartilage in the knee joint
metabolism the sum of all the physical and chemical processes by which living substance is formed and maintained and by which energy is made available for use by the organism
metacarpal referring to the part of the hand between the wrist and fingers
micturate (urinate, void) to pass urine from the body
midclavicular line an imaginary line that runs inferiorly and vertically from the center of the clavicle
midsternal line an imaginary line that runs vertically through the middle of the sternum
miosis constriction of the pupil
MMR combined measles, mumps, and rubella vaccine
mons pubis a pillow of adipose tissue situated over the symphysis pubis and covered by coarse hair; also called the *mons veneris*
Montgomery straps tie tapes used to hold dressings in place
morbidity incidence of disease
mucolytic destroying or dissolving mucus
mucous membrane epithelial tissue that lines passages and cavities communicating with the air
mucus a viscous fluid secreted by the mucous membranes
murmur (cardiac) abnormal sounds heard on auscultation of the heart resulting from turbulent blood flow during systole and diastole
mydriatic a medication that dilates the pupils
myelogram an x-ray film of the spinal cord, nerve roots, and vertebrae after injection of a contrast media into the subarachnoid space
myocardial infarction cardiac tissue necrosis resulting from obstruction of the blood flow to the heart
myocardium the heart muscle; the middle layer of the heart tissue
narcotic antagonist a drug that prevents or reverses the action of a narcotic
nasogastric tube a plastic or rubber tube inserted through the nose into the stomach
nasopharynx the upper part of the pharynx adjoining the nasal passage
nausea the urge to vomit
nebulizer an atomizer or sprayer
necrosis death of cells or tissue in contact with living cells
negative nitrogen balance a nitrogen output that exceeds nitrogen intake (related to protein balance)
neoplasm any growth that is new and abnormal

nephritis inflammation of a kidney
nephron the functional unit of the kidney
nephrosis a disease of the kidney in which there is degeneration of kidney function without inflammation; also called *nephrotic syndrome*
nerve block chemical interruption of a nerve pathway effected by injecting a local anesthetic
neurologic pertaining to the nervous system
nocturia (nycturia) increased frequency of urination at night
nocturnal enuresis involuntary urination at night
nonproductive cough a dry, harsh cough without secretions
normal saline an isotonic concentration of salt (NaCl) solution
nosocomial referring to or originating in a hospital or similar institution, as in a nosocomial infection
obesity weight that is 20% greater than the ideal for height and frame
objective data client information that can be determined by observation or measurement by laboratory studies or other means and that can be tested against an accepted standard
obturator anything that obstructs or closes an opening; the obturator of a tracheostomy set fits inside and closes off the end of the outer tube
ointment a semisolid preparation applied externally to the body
olfactory referring to the sense of smell
oliguria production of abnormally small amounts of urine by the kidneys
operative (intraoperative) period the time during surgery
ophthalmoscope an instrument used to examine the interior of the eye
opportunistic pathogen microorganism that causes disease only in a susceptible person
orientation awareness of time, place, and person
orifice an external opening of a body cavity; for example, the anus is the orifice of the large intestine
oropharynx the part of the pharynx that lies between the upper aspect of the epiglottis and the soft palate
orthopnea the ability to breathe only in the upright position, that is, sitting or standing
orthostatic hypotension decrease in blood pressure that occurs on assuming a sitting or standing position
osteoarthritis noninflammatory degenerative joint disease
osteoporosis decrease in bone density; demineralization of bone
ostomy a suffix denoting the formation of an opening or outlet
otoscope an instrument used to inspect the eardrum and external ear canal
outward rotation a turning away from the midline
overweight weight that is 10% greater than the ideal for height and frame
packing filling an open wound or cavity with a material such as gauze

$PaCO_2$ partial pressure of carbon dioxide (arterial blood)
palate the roof of the mouth
palliative affording relief without curing
pallor absence of normal skin color; a whitish-grayish tinge
palpation the act of feeling with the hands, usually the fingers
pandemic an epidemic disease that is widespread
PaO_2 partial pressure of oxygen (arterial blood)
papule a small, superficial, round elevation of the skin
paracentesis the insertion of a needle into a cavity (usually the abdominal cavity) to remove fluid
paradoxical breathing the ballooning out of the chest wall during expiration and depression or sucking inward of the chest wall during inspiration
paralysis the impairment or loss of motor function of a body part
paraplegia paralysis of the lower part of the body (including the legs) affecting both motor function and sensation
parasites plants or animals that live on or within another living organism
parenchyma the functional or essential elements of an organ
parenteral accomplished by a needle; occurring outside the alimentary tract; injected into the body through some route other than the alimentary canal, for example, intravenously
paresis partial or incomplete paralysis
paresthesia an abnormal sensation of numbness, burning, or prickling
paronychia inflammation of the tissue surrounding the nail
parotitis (parotiditis) inflammation of the parotid salivary gland
passive exercise exercise during which the muscles do not contract and the nurse, therapist, or client supplies the energy to move the client's body part
paste a semisolid dermatologic preparation that is applied externally
patent open, unobstructed, not closed
pathogen a microorganism capable of producing disease
PCO_2 partial pressure of carbon dioxide
peak plasma level (of drug) the concentration of a drug in the blood plasma that occurs when the elimination rate equals the rate of absorption
pediculosis infestation with lice
penetrating wound a wound created by an instrument that penetrated the skin or mucous membranes deeply into the tissues
Penrose drain a flexible rubber drain
percussion an assessment method in which the body surface is tapped or struck to elicit sound or vibrations from the body structures below the struck area
percutaneous electric stimulation stimulation of major peripheral nerves by electricity applied to the skin surface
perfusion passage of fluid through the vessels of an organ or tissue
perineum the area between the anus and the genitals

perioperative period the time before, during, and after an operation
periorbital around the eye socket
peripheral at the edge or outward boundary
peripheral pulse a pulse located in the periphery of the body
peristalsis wavelike movements produced by circular and longitudinal muscle fibers of the intestinal walls; it propels the intestinal contents onward
peristomal referring to the skin area that surrounds a stoma
peritoneal cavity the area between the layers of peritoneum in the abdomen; a potential space
peritoneum the membrane lining the abdominal walls
peritonitis inflammation of the peritoneum
perspiration the fluid secreted by the sweat glands for excreting waste products and cooling the body
petechiae pinpoint blood vessels visible on the skin
pH a measure of the relative alkalinity or acidity of a solution; a measure of the concentration of hydrogen ions
phalanx any bone of the fingers or toes (plural: phalanges)
phantom pain pain that remains after the perceived location has been removed, such as pain perceived in a foot after the leg has been amputated
phlebitis inflammation of a vein
phlebotomy opening a vein to remove blood
photosensitive sensitive to light
pitch the quality of sound based on the number of vibrations per second or the frequency of vibrations
pitting edema edema in which firm finger pressure on the skin produces an indentation (pit) that remains for several seconds
plantar flexion movement of the ankle so that the toes point downward
plasma the fluid portion of the blood in which the blood cells are suspended
pleural rub (friction rub) a coarse, leathery, or grating sound produced by the rubbing together of the pleura
pneumonia inflammation of the lung tissue
pneumothorax accumulation of air or gas in the pleural cavity
PO_2 partial pressure of oxygen (venous blood)
polydipsia excessive thirst
polyneuritis inflammation of many nerves
polyuria (diuresis) the production of abnormally large amounts of urine by the kidneys
popliteal referring to the posterior aspect of the knee
port an opening or entrance
posterior toward, or at the back of
postoperative (postsurgical) period the time following surgery
postural drainage drainage of secretions from various lung segments by the use of specific positions and gravity
precordium the area of the chest over the heart or lower thorax

preoperative period the time before an operation

prepuce see *foreskin*

primary intention healing wound healing that involves minimal or no tissue loss and in which there is minimal granulation tissue and scarring; also referred to as *primary union* or *first intention healing*

proctoscopy visualization of the interior of the rectum with a proctoscope

prodromal period the time from the onset of nonspecific symptoms to the appearance of specific symptoms

prognosis the medical opinion about the outcome of a disease

pronation turning the palm downward; moving the bones of the forearm so that the palm of the hand turns from anterior to posterior in the anatomic position

prone (prone position) lying on the abdomen with the face turned to one side

prophylaxis preventive treatment; prevention of disease

prostatectomy the removal of the prostate gland

prosthesis an artificial part, such as a glass eye, an artificial leg, or dentures

proteinuria the presence of protein in the urine

protocol written plan specifying the procedures to be followed in a particular situation

proximal closest to the point of attachment

pruritus intense itching

ptosis an eyelid that lies at or below the pupil margin; drooping

pulmonary embolus a blood clot that has moved to the lungs

pulse the wave of blood within an artery that is created by contraction of the left ventricle of the heart

pulse deficit a difference between the apical and the radial pulses

pulse pressure the difference between the systolic and the diastolic pressures

pulse rate the number of pulse beats per minute

pulse rhythm the pattern of pulse beats and of intervals between beats

pulse volume the force of the blood with each beat produced by contraction of the left ventricle; pulse strength

puncture (stab) wound a wound made by a sharp instrument penetrating the skin and underlying tissues

purulent containing pus

pus a thick liquid associated with inflammation and composed of cells, liquid, microorganisms, and tissue debris

pustule a small elevation of the skin or mucous membrane, or a clogged pore or follicle containing pus

putrid rotten

pyelogram an x-ray film of the kidney and ureter, showing the pelvis of the kidney

pyrexia elevated body temperature; fever

pyuria the presence of pus in the urine

quality (of sound) subjective description of a sound (e.g., whistling, gurgling, or snapping)

radial pulse the pulse point located where the radial artery passes over the radius of the arm

radiating pain pain perceived at the source and in surrounding or nearby structures

rales see *crackles*

range of motion (ROM) the degree of movement possible for each joint

rebound phenomenon (thermal) the time when the maximum therapeutic effect of a hot or cold application is achieved and the opposite effect begins

reconstitution the technique of adding a solvent to a powdered drug to prepare it for injection

referred pain pain perceived to be in one area but whose source is in another area

reflex an involuntary activity in response to a stimulus

reflux backward flow

regeneration the replacement of destroyed tissue cells by cells that are identical or similar in structure and function

regurgitation the spitting up or backward flow of undigested food

rehabilitation the restoration of a person who is ill or injured to the highest possible functional capacity

renal relating to the kidney

renal dialysis a process in which blood flows from an artery through an artificial membrane that removes impurities; the blood then returns to the client through a vein

renal pelvis the funnel-shaped upper end of each ureter

residual urine the amount of urine remaining in the bladder after a person voids

residual volume (air) the amount of air remaining in the lungs after a person exhales both tidal and expiratory reserve volumes

resonance a low-pitched, hollow sound produced over normal lung tissue when the chest is percussed

respiration the act of breathing; transport of oxygen from the atmosphere to the body cells and transport of carbon dioxide from the cells to the atmosphere

respiratory acidosis (hypercapnia) a state of excess carbon dioxide in the body

respiratory arrest the sudden cessation of breathing

resuscitate to restore life; to revive

retching the involuntary attempt to vomit without producing vomitus

retention (urinary) the accumulation of urine in the bladder and the inability of the bladder to empty itself

retrograde pyelogram an x-ray film taken after a contrast medium is injected through ureteral catheters into the kidneys

retroperitoneal behind the peritoneum

reverse isolation (barrier technique) measures used to prevent certain clients, such as those with severe burns, from coming in contact with microorganisms

reverse Trendelenburg's position a position with the head of the bed raised and the foot lowered, while the bed foundation remains even

Rh factor antigens present on the surface of some people's erythrocytes; persons who possess this factor are referred to as Rh positive, whereas those who do not are referred to as Rh negative

rhinitis inflammation of the mucous membrane of the nose

rhonchi coarse, dry, wheezy, or whistling sounds, more audible during exhalation as the air moves through tenacious mucus or a constricted bronchus

roentgenogram a film produced by photography with x-rays

rotation turning a bone around its central axis either toward the midline of the body (internal rotation) or away from the midline of the body (external rotation)

Salem sump tube a double-lumen nasogastric tube

sanguineous bloody

sanguineous exudate an exudate containing large amounts of red blood cells

saphenous vein either of two superficial veins of the legs; the greater one extends from the foot to the inguinal region, whereas the lesser one extends from the foot up the back of the leg to the knee joint

scar (cicatrix) tissue dense fibrous tissue derived from granulation tissue

sclerosis a process of hardening that occurs from inflammation and disease of the interstitial substance; the term is used to describe hardening of nervous tissues and arterioles

scoliosis a lateral curvature of a part of the vertebral column

sebaceous gland a gland of the dermis that secretes sebum

seborrheic dermatitis a chronic disease of the skin, characterized by scaling and crusted patches on various body areas, such as the scalp

secondary intention healing wound healing that involves the formation of extensive granulation tissue and in which the repair time is lengthy and scarring is extensive

secretion the product of a gland; for example, saliva is the secretion of the salivary glands

sedative an agent that tends to calm or tranquilize

semi-Fowler's position a bed-sitting position in which the head of the bed is elevated at least 30 degrees, with or without knee flexion; also referred to as low-Fowler's position

sensitivity quick response, often referring to the response of microorganisms to an antibiotic

septic referring to a disease process produced by microorganisms or to their poisonous products in the blood

serosanguineous composed of serum and blood
serous exudate a watery exudate composed mainly of serum
serum (blood) blood plasma from which the fibrinogen has been separated during clotting
shock acute circulatory failure
Sickle cell scythe-shaped erythrocytes; common to Mediterranean and African populations
side effect an unintended action or complication of a drug
sigmoidoscopy examination of the interior of the sigmoid colon with a sigmoidoscope
sitz bath (hip bath) bath used to soak a client's pelvic or perineal area
sleep apnea periodic cessation of breathing during sleep
smear material spread across a glass slide in preparation for microscopic study
spasm involuntary contraction of a muscle or muscle group
specific gravity the weight or degree of concentration of a substance compared with the weight of an equal amount of another substance used as a standard; for example, water used as a standard has a specific gravity of 1, whereas urine in comparison has a specific gravity of 1.010 to 1.025
speculum a funnel-shaped instrument used to widen and examine canals of the body, such as the vagina or nasal canal
sphincter a ringlike muscle that opens or closes a natural orifice (e.g., the urethra) when it relaxes or contracts
sphygmomanometer an instrument used to measure the pressure of the blood in the arteries
spirometry the measurement of pulmonary volumes and capacities using a spirometer
splint a rigid bar or appliance used to stabilize a body part
sprain injury of the ligaments and associated structure of a joint by wrenching or twisting; associated structures include tendons, muscles, nerves, and blood vessels
sputum the mucous secretion from the lungs, bronchi, and trachea that is expectorated through the mouth
stasis stagnation or stoppage of flow of body fluids, such as intestinal fluids, urine, or blood
stenosis constriction or narrowing of a body canal, vessel, or opening
sterile free from microorganisms, including spores
sterile technique see *surgical asepsis*
sterilization a process that destroys all microorganisms, including spores; causing inability to reproduce
stertor snoring or sonorous respiration, usually due to a partial obstruction of the upper airway
stethoscope an instrument used to listen to various sounds inside the body, such as the heartbeat
stoma an artificial opening; it may be permanent or temporary
stool (feces) waste products excreted from the large intestine

stopcock a valve that controls the flow of fluid or air through a tube
strain (of a muscle) overexertion or overstretching of a muscle or part of a muscle
stridor a shrill, harsh, crowing sound made on inhalation; due to constriction of the upper airway or laryngeal obstruction
stroke volume the amount of blood ejected from the heart with each ventricular contraction
stupor a condition of partial or nearly complete unconsciousness; stuporous clients are never fully awakened even when painfully stimulated
stylet a metal or plastic probe inserted into a needle or cannula to render it stiff and to prevent occlusion of the lumen by particles of tissue
subcostal below the ribs
subcutaneous (hypodermic) beneath the layers of the skin
subjective data client information that only the client can give, such as thoughts or feelings
sublingual under the tongue
suborbital beneath the orbit (the bony cavity containing the eyeball)
subscapular below the scapula (shoulder blade)
substernal retractions indrawing beneath the sternum (breastbone)
supination turning the palm upward; moving the bones of the forearm so that the palm of the hand turns from posterior to anterior in the anatomic position
supine (supine position) lying on the back with the face upward; also called *dorsal position*
suppository a solid, cone-shaped, medicated substance inserted into the rectum, vagina, or urethra
supraclavicular retractions indrawing above the clavicles (collarbones)
suprapubic above the pubic arch
suprasternal retractions indrawing above the sternum
surfactant a lipoprotein mixture secreted in the alveoli that reduces surface tension of the fluid lining the alveoli
surgical asepsis measures that render and maintain objects free of all microorganisms including spores (sterile)
suture in surgery, a surgical stitch used to close accidental or surgical wounds; in anatomy, a junction line of the skull bones
symptoms (covert data) see *subjective data*
syncope fainting or temporary loss of consciousness
syndrome a group of signs and symptoms resulting from a single cause and constituting a typical clinical picture, such as the shock syndrome
synovial joint a freely movable joint surrounded by a capsule enclosing a cavity that contains a transparent, viscid fluid
syphilis a sexually transmitted disease caused by the microorganism *Treponema pallidum*
syringe an instrument used to inject or withdraw liquids
systemic pertaining to the body (or other system) as a whole

systole the period when the ventricles of the heart are contracted

systolic pressure the pressure of the blood against the arterial walls when the ventricles of the heart contract

tablet a medication in solid form that is compressed and molded

tachycardia an excessively rapid pulse or heart rate, over 100 beats per minute in an adult

tachypnea abnormally fast respirations, usually more than 24 per minute, marked by quick, shallow breaths

tactile (vocal) fremitus vibrations, palpable with the palms of the hands, originating in the larynx and transmitted to the chest wall during speech

T-binder a cloth in the shape of a T often used to retain dressings in the genital region

Td combined tetanus and diphtheria toxoid used for people over 6 years of age; it has less diphtheria toxoid than does DT

temporal pulse a pulse point where the temporal artery passes over the temporal bone of the skull

tenesmus straining; painful, ineffective straining during defecation or urination

tetany a syndrome manifested by muscle twitching, cramps, convulsions, and sharp flexion of the wrist and ankle joints

therapy treatment or remedy

thrombocytopenia an abnormal reduction in the number of platelets in the blood

thrombophlebitis inflammation of a vein followed by formation of a blood clot

thrombosis the development of a blood clot

thrombus a solid mass of blood constituents in the circulatory system; a clot (plural: thrombi)

tic a repetitive twitching of the muscles, often of the face or upper trunk

tidal volume the volume of air that is normally inhaled and exhaled

tinnitus a ringing or buzzing sensation in the ears

tissue perfusion supplying nutrients and oxygen to body tissues and organs

tomography a scanning procedure during which several x-ray beams pass through the body part from different angles

tonicity the normal condition of tension or tone, for example, of a muscle

tonus the slight, continual contraction of muscles

topical applied externally, for example, to the skin or mucous membranes

tortuous twisted

total lung capacity the maximum volume to which the lungs can be expanded

total parenteral nutrition administration of a hypertonic solution of carbohydrates, amino acids, and lipids by an indwelling intravenous catheter placed into the superior vena cava via the jugular or subclavian vein; also called *intravenous hyperalimentation*

tourniquet a device, such as a rubber strip, that is wrapped around a body area to compress the blood vessels

toxemia a generalized toxic state caused by the distribution of poisonous products of bacteria throughout the body

toxin a poison produced by some microorganisms, animals, and plants

tracheal tug an indrawing and downward pulling of the trachea during inhalation

tracheostomy procedure by which an opening is made in the anterior portion of the trachea and a cannula is introduced into the opening

traction the exertion of a pulling force

trademark (brand name) name of drug given by the drug manufacturer

transcutaneous electrical nerve stimulation (TENS) the placement of electrodes on the surface of the skin over a peripheral nerve pathway for the purpose of relieving pain

transfusion the introduction of whole blood or its components, such as serum, erythrocytes, or platelets, into the venous circulation

trapeze bar a triangular handgrip suspended from an overbed frame

trauma injury

tremor an involuntary muscle contraction, for example, quivering, twitching, or convulsions

Trendelenburg's position a bed position with the head of the bed lowered and the foot raised, while the bed foundation remains even; in some agencies, the position involves elevation of the knees, with the feet lowered and the head lowered

trocar a sharp, pointed instrument that fits inside a cannula and is used to pierce body cavities

trochanter either of two processes below the neck of the femur

trochanter roll a rolled towel support placed against the hips to prevent external rotation of the legs

troche a lozenge

tumor an uncontrolled and progressive growth of cells

tuning fork an instrument shaped like a two-pronged fork and made of metal; the prongs vibrate when struck

turgor normal cell tension; fullness

tympany a hollow, drumlike sound produced on percussion over organs that contain gas or air

ulcer a localized sloughing of skin tissue or mucous membrane commonly associated with varicosities or hyperactivity of the gastrointestinal tract

ultrasound high-frequency, mechanical, radiant energy

unconscious incapable of responding to sensory stimuli; insensible

unilateral affecting one side

unit dose system (of drugs) prepackaged and labeled individual doses of medication for each client; the amount of medication the client is to receive at a prescribed hour

universal donor a person with type O blood

universal recipient a person with type AB blood

unsterile containing microorganisms; unsterile material may be clean or contaminated

urea a substance found in urine, blood, and lymph; the main nitrogenous substance in blood

ureterostomy an artificial opening into the ureter

urethritis inflammation of the urethra

urgency (urinary) a feeling that one must urinate

urinal a receptacle used to collect urine

urinalysis a laboratory analysis of the urine

urinary diversion see *urostomy*

urobilinogen a colorless compound found in the intestines from the reduction of bilirubin

urostomy (ureterostomy, urinary diversion) an opening through the abdominal wall into the urinary tract that permits the drainage of urine

urticaria an allergic reaction marked by smooth, reddened, slightly elevated patches of skin and intense itching (hives)

uvula a small fleshy mass projecting from the soft palate above the base of the tongue

vaccine suspension of killed, attenuated, or living microorganisms administered to prevent or treat an infectious disease

Valsalva maneuver forceful exhalation against a closed glottis, which increases intrathoracic pressure

varicosity the state of having swollen, distended, and knotted veins, especially in the legs

vasectomy ligation and cutting of the vas deferens, rendering the male sterile

vasoconstriction a decrease in the caliber (lumen) of blood vessels

vasodilation an increase in the caliber (lumen) of blood vessels

vasopressor an agent that causes the blood pressure to rise

vasospasm spasm or constriction of the blood vessels

ventilation the movement of air; the act of breathing

ventral toward or at the front of; anterior

ventricle a small cavity, such as those located in the brain or the heart

vertigo dizziness

vesicular sounds normal, quiet, rustling, or swishing respiratory sounds heard over the terminal bronchioles and alveoli during auscultation

vial a glass medication container with a sealed rubber cap, for single or multiple doses

vibration a technique of rapidly agitating the hands while pressing on a body area

virulence the degree of strength or power of an organism to produce disease

virus minute infectious agent smaller than a bacterium

viscera large interior organs in body cavities, such as the liver and stomach (singular: viscus)

viscosity the quality of being viscous; the thickness or resistance of a fluid

vital capacity maximum amount of air that can be exhaled following a maximum inhalation

vital (cardinal) signs measurement of physiological functioning—specifically, temperature, pulse, respirations, and blood pressure; may include pain and pulse oximetry

vitiligo patches of hypopigmented skin

vocal resonance vibrations of the larynx transmitted during speech through the respiratory system to the chest wall

void urinate, micturate

vomitus material vomited

walker a metal, rectangular frame used as an aid to ambulation

Weber's test a test that assesses bone conduction of sound

wheal see *bleb*

wheeze a whistling sound on exhalation that usually indicates narrowing of the bronchial air passages

xiphoid process the tip of the sternum

x-rays electromagnetic radiations with extremely short wavelengths (Roentgen rays)

INDEX

Page numbers followed by *f* indicate figures; numbers followed by *t* indicate tables; numbers followed by *b* indicate boxes.

A
Abbreviations
  common, 164–165
  "do not use" abbreviations, 166–167
Abbreviations
  medication orders, 128t
Abdomen
  abdominal distention, 101
  adults, older, 57–58
  physical health examination, 47, 48f
Abdominal (diaphragmatic) breathing, 227
Abduction, 221
ABGs. *See* arterial blood gases (ABGs)
Abrasion, defined, 221
Abscess, 221
Absorption (of drug), 221
Acetone in urine, 97
Acid-fast bacilli (AFB) test, 197
Acidosis (acidemia), 221
Acromion (acromial process), 221
Actinic keratoses, 52
Activities of daily living (ADLs), 221
Acute, defined, 221
Adduction, 221
ADH (antidiuretic hormone), 222
Adipose, defined, 221
Adults, older
  communication guidelines
    common problems, 13
    elderspeak, characteristics of, 12–13
    interventions to improve, 13–14
  fecal elimination, 103
  fluid and electrolyte balance, 82–83
  medication administration, 127, 129
  pain, 87
  physical health examination
    abdomen, breasts, and axillae, 57–58
    cardiovascular and peripheral vascular systems, 56–57
    ears and hearing, 54
    eyes and vision, 53
    genitals, 60
    hair, 52
    history, 51
    mouth, 54–55
    musculoskeletal system, 58
    nails, 52
    neurologic system, 58–60
    nose and sinuses, 54
    skin, 51–52
    thorax and lungs, 55–56
  pressure areas, 107, 110
  respiratory function, 91
  teaching and learning, 123–124
  tube feedings, 95
  urinary elimination, 99–100
  wounds, healing, 115
Adventitious breath sounds
  defined, 221
Adventitious breath sounds
  described, cause, and location, 44t
Aerosol (inhalation) therapy, 233
AFB (acid-fast bacilli) test, 197
Airborne precautions, 158
Alanine amino transferase (ALT), 184t
Albumin blood levels
  hypoalbuminemia, 232
  normal findings and clinical implications, 184t

Alcoholism, 23
Aldosterone, 221
Alginate dressings, 113t
Alkaline phosphatase levels, 185t
Alkalosis (alkalemia), 221
Allergies
  anaphylaxis, 221
  family history, 23
  past history, 23
Alopecia, 221
ALT (alanine amino transferase), 184t
American Association of Critical Care Nurses, 14–15
American Nurses Association Code of Ethics, 144
Ammonia blood levels, 185t
Ampule, defined, 221
Analgesic, defined, 221
Anaphylaxis (anaphylactic shock, anaphylactic reaction), 221
Anemia, 221
Anesthesia, 221
Aneurysm, 221
Angiography
  defined, 222
  nursing interventions, 209t
Angry clients, 7
Anorexia, 222
Anoscopy, 202t
Anterior, defined, 222
Anterior thorax, examination of, 43–45, 43t, 44t
Antibiotic, 222
Antibody (immunoglobulin), defined, 222, 232
Antidiuretic hormone (ADH), 222
Antigen, 222
Antipyretic, 222
Antiseptic, 222
Anuria, 222
Anus
  anoscopy, 202t
  examination of, 51
Anxious clients, 9–10
Aphasia
  communication guidelines, 11
  defined, 222
Apical pulse, 222
Apical-radial pulse, 222
APIE (Assessment, Plan, Implementation, Evaluation) documentation format, 149, 150–151f
Apnea
  defined, 222
  respiratory function, 89
Apothecaries system of measurement, 176–177
Appearance of the client, 37
Approximate, defined, 222
Arcus senilis, 53
Arrhythmia, 222
Arterial blood gases (ABGs)
  fluid and electrolyte balance, 79
  purpose of, 197
  respiratory function, 89
Arterial blood gases (ABGs)
  normal findings and clinical implications, 193t
Arteriosclerosis, 222
Arthritis
  family history, 23
  osteoarthritis, defined, 237
Ascites, 222
Ascorbic acid (vitamin C), 214t
Asepsis, 222
Asphyxia, 222
Aspirate, defined, 222
Assessing, as component of nursing process, 2
Assessment and diagnosis
  examination methods, 28–29
  nursing diagnoses
    formulating diagnostic statements, 61–62
    NANDA-approved nursing diagnoses, 62–68
  nursing health history, 22–27
  physical examination
    abdomen, 47, 48f, 57–58
    breasts and axillae, 46–47, 57
    cardiovascular and peripheral vascular system, 45–46, 46f, 56–57
    female genitals and inguinal lymph nodes, 50, 60
    general survey, 37–38
    head, 39–42, 53–55
    integumentary system, 38, 51–52
    male genitals and inguinal area, 50–51, 60
    musculoskeletal system, 48–49, 58
    neurologic system, 49–50, 58–60
    older adults, special considerations for, 51–60
    preparing the client, 36–37
    rectum and anus, 51
  vital signs, 30–35, 32f
Assessment and diagnosis
  physical examination
    thorax and lungs, 42–45, 43t, 44t, 55–56

AST (aspartate amino transferase), 184t
Astringent, 222
Ataxia, 222
Atelectasis
  defined, 222
  postoperative period, 117
Atony, 222
Atrophy, 222
Auricles, examination of, 40
Auscultation. *See also* breath sounds
  abdomen, of, 47, 48f
  chest, 89
  defined, 222
  examination method, 29
Auscultation
  lungs, 43, 43t, 44t, 45
Axilla
  defined, 222
  physical health examination, 47
Axillary line, 222

B

Bacteriuria, 222
Balance test, 49
Barium, defined, 222
Barium enema. *See also* lower gastrointestinal (LGI) tests
  defined, 223
  nursing interventions, 204t
Barium swallow
  defined, 223
  nursing interventions, 203t
Barrel chest, 223
Barrier technique (reverse isolation), 242
Basal metabolic rate (BMR), 223
Basic formula method of dosage calculation, 129
Basophils, 182t
Bathrooms, hazards in, 74
Bedrooms, hazards in, 74
Bilateral, defined, 223
Bile duct studies
  cholangiogram, 224
Bile duct studies
  IV cholangiogram, 206t, 236
  percutaneous transhepatic cholangiography, 207t
  postoperative cholangiography, 207t
Bilirubin
  blood levels, 185t
  defined, 223
  urine levels, 194t
Binder, defined, 223
Biographic data for nursing health history, 22
Biopsy, 223
Biotin, 214t
Bladder, examination of, 47
Bleb (wheal), 223
Bleeding
  family history, 23
  postoperative period, 116
Blood (serum)
  defined, 243
  urine, in, 97, 230
Blood pressure
  fluid and electrolyte balance, 78
  hypertension, 23, 231
  hypotension, 232
  orthostatic hypotension, 237
  postoperative period, 116
  procedure for taking, 33–34
Blood tests. *See under* laboratory tests
Blood urea nitrogen (BUN)
  blood levels, and urinary elimination, 98
  purpose of, 197
Bloodborne pathogens
  diseases transmitted, 160
  postexposure prophylaxis, 161–162
  steps to follow after exposure, 160–161
BMR (basal metabolic rate), 223
BNP (brain natriuretic peptide) level, 188t
Body mechanics, principles of, 71–72
Body temperature. *See also* fever
  core temperature, 225
  fluid and electrolyte balance, 78
  hypothermia, 232
  methods for assessment, 30
  postoperative period, 116
  range for, 31
Bolus (intravenous push, IVP), 234
Bones, examination of, 48
Bowel sounds, 101
Brachial pulse, 223
Braden Scale for Predicting Pressure Sore Risk, 107, 108–109f
Bradycardia, 223
Bradypnea, 89
Brain natriuretic peptide (BNP) level, 188t
Brand name (trademark), 250
Breasts
  examination of, in older adults, 57
  physical health examination, 46–47
  review of, for nursing health history, 26
Breath sounds
  abnormal, 89–90
  adventitious, defined, 221

Breath sounds
adventitious, 44t
normal, 42t
Breathing patterns, abnormal, 89
Bronchial sounds, 43t, 223
Bronchodilator, 223
Bronchopneumonia, 223
Bronchoscope
defined, 223
nursing interventions, 199–200t
Bronchovesicular sounds, 43t, 223
Bruxism, 223
B-type natriuretic peptide, 188t
Bubbling respirations, 90
Buccal, defined, 223
Buccal mucosa, 41
Buffer, defined, 223
Bulimia, 223
BUN. *See* blood urea nitrogen (BUN)

C

C. difficile, 159
Calciferol (vitamin D), 211t
Calcium
blood levels, 191t, 231, 232
hypercalcemia, 231
hypercalciuria, 231
hypocalcemia, 232
information about, 215t
urine, in, 194t, 231
Calculus, defined, 223
Cancer, family history of, 23
Cannula, 223
Canthus, 223
Carbon dioxide, 238
Cardiac arrest, 223
Cardiac output, 223
Cardinal signs. *See* vital (cardinal) signs
Cardiopulmonary resuscitation (CPR), 223
Cardiovascular system
circulatory overload, defined, 224
circulatory system, root words for, 168
compliance (vascular), 225
CPR, 224
examination, in older adults, 56–57
physical health examination, 45, 46f
review of, for nursing health history, 26
Cardiovascular system
blood tests, 186–188t
Caries, 224
Carina, defined, 224
Carminative, 224
Carotid arteries, 224
Cataract, 224
Cathartic (laxative), 224, 235
Catheter, defined, 224
Catheters, urinary
insertion of, 98
retention, removal of, 99
Caudal anesthetic, 224
Caviar spots, 55
CBC. *See* complete blood count (CBC)
Cellulitis, 224
Centigrade (Celsius), 224
Central venous pressure (CVP), 224
Central vessels, examination of, 45
Cephalocaudal, defined, 224
Cerebrospinal fluid, 224
Cerumen, 224
Chancre, 224
Change-of-shift reports, 18–29
Charting
guidelines for, 145
things to avoid, 145–146
Chest examination. *See also* lungs
auscultation, 89
chest movements, abnormal, 90
palpation, 88
percussion, 88
Chest roentgenogram (CXR), 198
Cheyne-Stokes respirations, 89, 224
Chickenpox, 23
Chief complaint, in nursing health history, 22
Chill, defined, 224
Chloride level
dietary sources, functions, and imbalances, 215t
normal findings and clinical implications, 191t
Cholangiogram, defined, 224. *See also* bile duct studies
Cholecystogram
defined, 224
Cholecystogram
nursing interventions, 205t
Cholesterol
defined, 224
hyperlipidemia, 231
Cholesterol
lipoprotein profile, 188–189t
Chromium, 217t
Chronic, defined, 224
Chyme, 224
Cicatrix (scar tissue), 224, 242
Cilia, 224
Circulatory overload, defined, 224
Circulatory system, 168. *See also* cardiovascular system

Circumduction, 224
CK (creatine kinase) level, 186t
Clean technique, 224
Cleansing enemas, 102
Clear absorbent acrylic dressings, 112t
Client assessment
  fluid and electrolyte balance
    history, 77
    laboratory tests, 78–79
    signs of imbalance, 78
    weight and vital signs, 78
  postoperative period, 116–117
  pressure areas, 103–106, 105f
  respiratory function, 87–88
  tube feedings, 91–92
  urinary elimination, 96–98
  wounds, healing, 114
Client information, essential, for documentation, 146–147
Clients, handling and moving, 72–73
Clinical guidelines
  clients with pain, individualizing care for, 83–87
  fecal elimination, 100–103
  fluid and electrolyte balance, 77–83
  healing wounds, 114–115
  postoperative period, 116–118
  pressure areas, 103–113, 105f, 108–109f, 111–113t
  respiratory function, 87–91
  tube feedings, 91–95
  urinary elimination, 96–100
Closed wound, 225
Clubbing (of nails), 225
Coagulate, defined, 225
Cobalamin (vitamin B_{12}), 213t
Cobalt, 217t
Cochlea, 225
Cognitive-behavioral modalities, and pain, 85–86
Colic, 225
Collagen, defined, 225
Collagen dressings, 112t
Colon cancer, 58
Colonoscope
  defined, 225
  nursing interventions, 202t
Colostomy, 225
Comatose, defined, 225
Commode, 225
Communicable disease (infectious disease), 225
Communication guidelines
  angry clients, 8
  anxious clients, 9–10
  confused clients, 8–9
  cultural issues, 11–12
  health professionals, communication among, 14–20
  importance of, 7
  language barriers, communicating across, 10–11
  older adults, 12–14
Complete blood count (CBC)
  purpose of, 197
  respiratory function, 89
Complete blood count (CBC)
  components and clinical implications, 179–183t
Compliance (vascular), 225
Computer records, and confidentiality, 144–145
Confidentiality, 144–145
Confused clients, communication with, 8–9
Congenital, defined, 225
Conjunctiva, 225
Conjunctivitis, 225
Consciousness, defined, 225. *See also* level of consciousness
Consensual reaction (of the eyes), 225
Constipation, 225
Contact precautions, 159
Contaminated, defined, 225
Contracture, defined, 225
Contusion, 225
Coping, facilitating, and pain, 86
Copper, 217t
Core temperature, 225
Cornea, 225
Cortisol (hydrocortisone), 233
Costal angle, 225
Costal (thoracic) breathing, 225
Costovertebral angle, 225
Coughs, 90
Counterirritant, defined, 225
Covert data (symptoms). *See* subjective data
CPR (cardiopulmonary resuscitation), 223
Crackles (rales)
  defined, 225
  described, cause, and location, 44t
  respiratory function, assessing, 90
Creatine kinase (CK) level, 186t
Creatinine
  blood levels, 98, 197
  defined, 226
Creatinine
  urine levels, 194t
Creatinine clearance in urine, 194t
Credé's maneuver, 226
Crepitus (crepitation), 226

Cultural issues and communication, 11–12
Culture, defined (microbiology), 226
Culture and sensitivity
  sputum, 197
  urine, 198
CVP (central venous pressure), 224
CXR (chest roentgenogram), 198
Cyanosis, 226
Cyst, 226
Cystitis, 226
Cystoscope, defined, 226
Cystoscopy
  defined, 226
Cystoscopy
  nursing interventions, 201t
Cytologic tests on sputum, 197
Cytology, defined, 226

D

Damp-to-damp dressings, 115
DAR (Data, Action, Response) (focus charting), 149, 152
Debride, defined, 226
Defecation, 226
Dehiscence
  defined, 226
  postoperative period, 118
Dehydration, 226
Delegation
  five "rights" of, 4
  principles for delegation to unlicensed personnel, 5–6
Delegation
  tasks for unlicensed personnel, examples of, 5t
Deltoid muscle for intramuscular injections, 139f, 140f
Dementia, 226
Dependent edema, 226
Dermatitis, 226
Dermatologic preparation, 226
Dermis (corium), 226
Detrusor muscle, 226
Dextrose, defined, 226. *See also* glucose
Diabetes, family history of, 23
Diagnosing, as nursing process component, 2
Diagnosis, defined, 226
Diagnostic statements
  three-part, 61–63
  two-part, 61
Diagnostic studies. *See also* laboratory tests; urinalysis; specific tests
  blood tests, 197
  cardiac tests, 198
  radiologic tests, 198
  sputum tests, 89, 197
  stool tests, 198
  tuberculin tests, 198
  urine tests, 198
Diaphoresis, 226
Diaphragmatic (abdominal) breathing, 226
Diarrhea, 226
Diastole, defined, 226
Diastolic pressure, 226
Differential count, 181–182t
Digestive system, root words for, 168–169
Digital, defined, 226
Dimensional analysis method of dosage calculation, 133–135
Diphtheria, 158
Direct percussion, as examination method, 29
Disorientation, 226
Distal, defined, 227
Distraction, for pain relief, 85
Diuresis
  defined, 227
  polyuria, 239
Diuretic, 228
"Do Not Use" abbreviations, 166–167
Documentation
  charting guidelines, 145–146
  confidentiality of computer records, 144–145
  essential client information, 146–147
  ethical and legal considerations, 144
  formats for
    focus charting (DAR), 149, 152
    narrative, 148–149
  formats for
    SOAP, SOAPIE, SOAPIER, and APIE, 149, 150–151f
Dorsal, defined, 227
Dorsal flexion, 227
Dorsal recumbent position, 227
Dorsalis pedis pulse, 227
Dosage calculation
  basic formula, 129
  dimensional analysis method, 133–135
  fractional equation method, 132–133
  ratio and proportion method, 132
  rounding numbers, 130–131
Drainage, defined, 228
Drainage tube patency, 116
Dressings
  wounds, for, 111–113t
  wounds, healing, 114–115

Droplet precautions, 158
Drug interaction, 227
Drug tolerance, 227
Drug toxicity, 227
Drug-resistant *enterococci,* 159
Dry sterile dressings, 114
Dullness (in percussion), 227
Dumping syndrome, 92
Duodenoscopy, 200t
Dysmenorrhea, 227
Dyspepsia, 227
Dysphagia, 227
Dysphoria, 227
Dyspnea
  defined, 227
  respiratory function, 89
Dysrhythmia, 227
Dysuria, 227

E

Ears
  older adults, examination of, 54
  physical health examination, 40
  review of, for nursing health history, 26
Ecchymosis, 227
ECF (extracellular fluid), 228
ECG. *See* electrocardiogram (ECG, EKG)
Edema, 227
EKG. *See* electrocardiogram (ECG, EKG)
Elderspeak, characteristics of, 12–13
Electrical hazards in the home, 74
Electrocardiogram (ECG, EKG)
  defined, 227
  purpose of, 198
Electroencephalogram, 227
Electrolytes
  defined, 227
  levels, and fluid and electrolyte balance, 78
  testing, purpose of, 197
Electrolytes
  normal findings and clinical implications, 190–192t
Embolus
  defined, 227
  postoperative period, 117
Emollient, 227
Emphysema, 227
Emulsion, 227
Endocrine system, for nursing health history, 27
Endogenous, defined, 227
Endoscope, defined, 227
Endoscopic examinations
  anoscopy, proctoscopy, sigmoidoscopy, and colonoscopy, 202t
  cystoscopy, 201t
  esophagoscopy, gastroscopy, and duodenoscopy, 200t
  laryngoscopy or bronchoscopy, 199–200t
Endothelium, 227
Endotracheal tube, 227
Enema
  cleansing enemas, 102
  defined, 228
  retention enemas, 103
Enteric, defined, 228
Enteric coated, defined, 228
Enteric feeding, 228
Enterostomal therapist, 228
Enzyme, 228
Eosinophils, 182t
Epidemic, defined, 228
Epidermis, 228
Epistaxis, 228
Eructation, 228
Erythema, 228
Erythrocyte, defined, 228
Eschar
  defined, 228
  pressure ulcers, 106
Esophagoscopy
  defined, 228
  nursing interventions, 200t
Ethical issues, and documentation, 144
Etiology
  defined, 228
  diagnostic statements, in, 61, 62
Eupnea, 228
Evaluation phase of nursing process
  components of, 153
  conclusions drawn from, 153–154
  nursing process component, 3
Evisceration
  defined, 228
  postoperative period, 118
Examination methods. *See also* individual methods
  auscultation, 29
  inspection, 28
  palpation, 28
  percussion, 28–29
Exanthema, 228
Excise, 228
Excoriation, 228
Excretion, 228
Exercise stress test, 198
Exogenous, defined, 228
Expectorate, 228

Expiratory reserve volume, 228
Extension, defined, 228
External cardiac massage, 228
Extracellular, defined, 228
Extracellular fluid (ECF), 228
Extraocular muscle tests, 40
Extravasation, 228
Exudate, 228
Eyes
  older adults, examination of, 53
  physical health examination, 39–40
  review of, for nursing health history, 26

F

Face, examination of, 39
Falls, preventing in health care agencies, 73–74
Family history of illness, 23
Fasting blood sugar, 197
Fat-soluble vitamins, 211–212t
Febrile, 228
Fecal elimination
  bowel sounds, 101
  client assessment, 100–102
  enemas, administering, 102–103
  older adults, special care for, 103
  postoperative period, 117, 118
  problems, risk factors for, 102
  vital signs, 101
Fecal impaction, 228
Fecal incontinence, 228
Feces (stool)
  consistency and color of, 101
  defined, 228, 248
  tests on, 198
Females
  genitourinary system, review of, for nursing health history, 27
  genitourinary system and inguinal area, examination of, 50
  genitourinary system assessment in older adults, 60
  mammography, 235
  reproductive system, root words for, 169
Femoral pulse, 228
Fever
  defined, 229
  hyperpyrexia, 231
  hyperthermia, 232
  pyrexia, 240
Fibrillation, 229
Fine motor tests, 49–50
Fire hazards
  A, B, C categories, 75
  fire extinguishers, using, 76
  homes, appraising for, 75
  RACE protocol, 75
First intention healing, 229, 240
Fistula, 229
Flaccid, defined, 229
Flaccid paralysis, 229
Flail chest, 229
Flatness (in percussion), 229
Flatulence
  defined, 229
  fecal elimination, 101
Flatus, 229
Flexion, defined, 229
Floor hazards, 74
Flowsheet, defined, 229
Fluid and electrolyte balance
  client assessment
    history, 77
    laboratory tests, 78–79
    signs of imbalance, 78
    weight and vital signs, 78
  fluid intake, restricting, 81–82
  imbalance, risks for, 79
  intake and output, monitoring, 78, 79–80
  normal or increased fluid intake, facilitating, 80–81
  older adults, special care for, 82–83
Fluid balance, during postoperative period, 116
Fluid intake
  normal or increased, facilitating, 80–81
  restricting, 81–82
Fluoride, 217t
Fluoroscope, 229
Flushing (of the skin), 229
Focus charting (DAR, Data, Action, Response), 149, 152
Folic acid (folate), 213t
Food tolerance during postoperative period, 117
Footdrop, 229
Forceps, 229
Foreskin, 229
Formulary, 229
Fowler's position, 229
Fractional equation method of dosage calculation, 132–133
Fracture, 229
Fremitus, 229
Frenulum, 229
Friction rub (pleural rub)
  defined, 229, 239
Friction rub (pleural rub)
  adventitious breath sound, 44t
Fundamental nursing

communication guidelines
angry clients, 8
anxious clients, 9–10
confused clients, 8–9
cultural issues, 11–12
health professionals, communication among, 14–20
importance of, 7
language barriers, communicating across, 10–11
older adults, 12–14
nursing process, components of, 2–3
Fundamental nursing
delegation, aspects of, 4–6, 5t
Furniture hazards, 74

G

Gait, 229
Gallbladder studies, 205t, 224
Gamma-glutamyl transferase (GGT), 186t
Gastric, defined, 229
Gastrocolic reflex, 229
Gastroenteritis, 229
Gastrointestinal suction, 118
Gastrointestinal system
older adults, examination of, 57–58
review of, for nursing health history, 26–27
Gastrointestinal tract studies
barium swallow, 203t, 222
lower GI series (barium enema), 204t, 223
upper GI series, 198, 203t
Gastroscopy
defined, 229
Gastroscopy
nursing interventions, 200t
Gastrostomy
defined, 229
tube feedings, 94–95
Gauge (of a needle), 230
Gavage, defined, 230
General health, review of, for nursing health history, 25
General survey
appearance, 37
mental status, 37–38
Generic name, 231
Genitourinary system. *See also* females; males
examination of, in older adults, 60
physical health examination, 50–51
review of, for nursing health history, 27
German measles. *See* rubella (German measles)
GGT (gamma-glutamyl transferase), 186t
Gingivitis, 230
Glans penis, 230
Glaucoma, 230
Glomerular filtrate, 230
Glossitis, 230
Glottis, 230
Glucose
defined, 230
dextrose, defined, 226
fasting blood levels, 197
hyperglycemia, 231
hypoglycemia, 232
urine, in, 97, 194t, 230
Glucose tolerance test (GTT), 197
Glycogen, 230
Glycosuria, 230
Gonorrhea, 230
Gout, 230
Granulation tissue, 230
GTT (glucose tolerance test), 197
Guaiac test, 198
Gums
adults, older, 54–55
physical health examination, 41
Gurgles. *See* rhonchi (gurgles)

H

Hair
adults, older, 52
physical health examination, 38
review of, for nursing health history, 26
Half-life (of drug), 230
Halitosis, 230
Hallux valgus, 230
Handoff communication, guidelines for, 17
Hct. *See* hematocrit (Hct)
HDL-C (high-density lipoprotein cholesterol), 189t
Head
physical health examination, 39–42
review of, for nursing health history, 26
Health care patterns, for nursing health history, 25
Health Insurance Portability and Accountability Act (HIPAA), 144
Health professionals, communication among
communication skills, elements of, 14–15
handoff communication/change-of-shift report, 17–19

Health professionals, communication among (*continued*)
SBAR guidelines, 15–17
telephone and verbal orders, 19–20
Hearing
adults, older, 54
physical health examination, 40
Hearing acuity tests, 40
Hearing-impaired clients, communication with, 11
Heart, examination of, 45, 46f
Heart disease, family history of, 23
Heimlich maneuver, 230
Hemangioma, 230
Hematemesis, 230
Hematocrit (Hct)
defined, 230
fluid and electrolyte balance, 78
Hematocrit (Hct)
normal findings and clinical implications, 180t
Hematoma, 230
Hematuria, 230
Hemiplegia, 230
Hemoglobin (Hgb)
defined, 230
normal findings and clinical implications, 179t
urine, in, 195t, 230
Hemoglobinuria, 230
Hemolysis, 230
Hemopneumothorax, 230
Hemoptysis, 90, 230
Hemorrhage, defined, 230
Hemorrhoids, 230
Hemothorax, 231
Heparin
defined, 231
site, needles, syringes, amount, and angle for injection, 142t
Heparin lock, 231
Hepatitis A, contact precautions for, 159
Hepatitis B virus
bloodborne pathogen, 160
postexposure prophylaxis, 162
Hepatitis C virus
bloodborne pathogen, 160
postexposure prophylaxis, 162
Hernia, 231
Hesitancy (of urination), 231
Hgb. *See* hemoglobin (Hgb)
High Fowler's position, 231
High-density lipoprotein cholesterol (HDL-C), 189t
Hip bath (sitz bath), 243
HIPAA (Health Insurance Portability and Accountability Act), 144
Hirsutism, 231
History. *See also* nursing health history
adults, older, 51
fluid and electrolyte balance, 77
respiratory function, 87–88
urinary elimination, 96
History of present illness, 22–23
HIV. *See* human immunodeficiency virus (HIV)
Homan's sign, 231
Homeostasis, 231
Homes
hazard appraisal, 74–75
infection control, 163
Household system of measurement, 177
Human immunodeficiency virus (HIV)
bloodborne pathogen, 160
postexposure prophylaxis, 161–162
Humidifier, defined, 231
Hydration, defined, 231
Hydrocephalus, 231
Hydrocolloid dressings, 111t
Hydrocortisone (cortisol), 231
Hydrogel dressings, 112t
Hyperalgesia, 231
Hyperalimentation, 231
Hypercalcemia, 231
Hypercalciuria, 231
Hypercapnia (respiratory acidosis), 231, 241
Hypercarbia (hypercapnia), 231, 241
Hyperemia, 231
Hyperextension, 231
Hyperglycemia, 231
Hyperhidrosis, 231
Hyperkalemia, 231
Hyperlipidemia, 231
Hypermagnesemia, 231
Hypernatremia, 231
Hyperplasia, defined, 231
Hyperpnea, 231
Hyperpyrexia, 231
Hyperreflexia, 231
Hyperresonance, 231
Hypersensitivity, 231
Hypersomnia, 231
Hypertension
defined, 231
family history, 23
Hyperthermia, 232
Hypertonic solution, 232
Hypertonicity, 232
Hypertrophy, 232
Hyperventilation, 89, 232
Hypervolemia, 232

Hypnotic (drug), 232
Hypoalbuminemia, 232
Hypocalcemia, 232
Hypodermic (subcutaneous), defined, 244. *See also* subcutaneous injections
Hypoglycemia, 232
Hypokalemia, 232
Hypomagnesemia, 232
Hyponatremia, 232
Hypoproteinemia, 232
Hypostatic pneumonia, 232
Hypotension, 232
Hypothermia, 232
Hypotonic solution, 232
Hypotonicity, 232
Hypoventilation, 89, 232
Hypovolemia, 232
Hypovolemic shock, 232
Hypoxemia, 232
Hypoxia, 232

I

Iatrogenic, 232
ICF (intracellular fluid), 233
Ileal conduit, 232
Ileostomy, 232
Immobility, 232
Immunity, 232
Immunizations
  defined, 232
  past history, 23
Immunoglobulin (antibody), defined, 222, 232
Impaction, 233
Impetigo, 159
Implementing, as nursing process component, 3
Impregnated nonadherent dressings, 111t
Incentive spirometer (sustained maximal inspiration [SMI] device), 233
Incision, defined, 233
Incompatibility (of drug), 233
Incontinence, 233
Incubation period, 233
Indirect percussion, as examination method, 29
Induration, 233
Infarct, 233
Infection, defined, 233
Infection control
  airborne precautions, 158
  bloodborne pathogens, 160–162
  contact precautions, 159
  droplet precautions, 158
  standard precautions, 156–157
  strategies for, 162–163
  transmission-based precautions, 157–159
Infectious disease (communicable disease), 225
Infiltration, defined, 233
Inflammation, 233
Infusion, defined, 233
Inguinal area, examination of, 50, 51
Inhalation (aerosol) therapy, 233
Injections
  rounding numbers, 131
  techniques for, 135
Injections
  subcutaneous, 137f, 142t
  intradermal, 136f, 142t
  intramuscular, 138–140f, 141f, 142t
Insomnia, 233
Inspection
  defined, 233
  examination method, 28
Instillation, 233
Insulin
  defined, 233
  site, needles, syringes, amount, and angle for injection, 142t
Intake and output, monitoring, 78, 79–80
Integument, defined, 233
Integumentary system, examination of, 38
Intercostal, defined, 233
Intercostal retractions, 90, 233
Internal rotation, 233
Interstitial, defined, 233
Interstitial fluid, 233
Intestinal distention, 233
Intracellular, defined, 233
Intracellular fluid (cellular fluid, ICF), 233
Intractable pain, 233
Intradermal (intracutaneous), defined, 233
Intradermal injections
  sites for, 136f
Intradermal injections
  sites, needles, syringes, mounts, angles, 142t
Intramuscular, defined, 233
Intramuscular injections
  sites for, 138–140f
  Z-track method, 141f
Intramuscular injections
  sites, needles, syringes, mounts, angles, 142t

Intraoperative (operative) period, 233, 237
Intrapleural, defined, 233
Intrathecal, defined, 234
Intravascular, defined, 234
Intravenous, defined, 234
Intravenous cholangiogram
  defined, 234
Intravenous cholangiogram
  nursing interventions, 206t
Intravenous hyperalimentation (total parenteral nutrition), 245
Intravenous (IV) infusions
  postoperative period, 116
  rounding numbers, 131
Intravenous push (IVP, bolus), 234
Intravenous pyelogram, defined, 234
Intravenous pyelography (IVP)
  defined, 234
Intravenous pyelography (IVP)
  nursing interventions, 208t
Intravenous urography (IVU)
  defined, 234
Intravenous urography (IVU)
  nursing interventions, 208t
Intravertebral (intraspinal), defined, 234
Intubated clients, communication with, 11
Intubation, defined, 234
Inversion, defined, 234
Iodine, 218t
Ion, defined, 234
Iron, 218t
Iron-deficiency anemia, 234
Irradiation, 234
Irrigation (lavage)
  defined, 234, 235
  postoperative period, 118
Irritant, 234
Ischemia, 234
Isolation, 234
Isometric, 234
Isotonic, 234
IVP. *See* intravenous pyelography (IVP)
IVP (intravenous push, bolus), 234

J

Jaundice, 234
Jejunostomy tube feedings, 94–95
Jejunum, 234
Joints, examination of, 49

K

Kardex, 234
Kegel's exercises, 234
Ketone bodies in urine, 195t
Ketosis, 234
Kinesthetic sensation, examination of, 50
Kitchen hazards, 74
Korotkoff's sounds, 234
Kyphosis, 55, 234

L

Laboratory tests. *See also* diagnostic studies; specific laboratory tests
  blood
    common diagnostic, purpose of, 197
  fluid and electrolyte balance, 78–79
  respiratory function, 89
  sputum, 89, 197
  urine, on, 97–98
  variation among agencies, 178
Laboratory tests
  blood
    arterial blood gases, 79, 89, 193t, 197
    chemistry tests, 184–189t
    complete blood count, 179–183t
    electrolytes, 190–192t
    serum osmolality, 192t
  urine, on, 194–195t
Labored breathing, 234
Lacerate, defined, 234
Lacrimal sac, 234
Lacrimation, 235
Language barriers, 10–11
Laryngeal stridor, 235
Laryngoscopy
  defined, 235
  nursing interventions, 199–200t
Laryngospasm, 235
Lateral, defined, 235
Lateral position, 235
Lavage (irrigation)
  defined, 236, 235
  postoperative period, 118
Laxative (cathartic), 224, 235
LDL (low-density lipoprotein), 189t
Learning. *see* teaching and learning
Legal issues, with documentation, 144
Lentigo senilis, 235
Lesion, 235
Lethargy, 235
Leukocyte
  defined, 235
Leukocyte
  WBC count with differential, 181–182t
Leukocytosis, 235

Level of consciousness
consciousness, defined, 225
postoperative period, 116
unconscious, defined, 246
Levin tube, 235
LGI tests. *See* lower gastrointestinal (LGI) tests
Lifestyle, for nursing health history, 24
Ligament, 235
Liniment, 235
Lipoprotein profile
cholesterol, defined, 224
hyperlipidemia, 231
Lipoprotein profile
normal findings and clinical implications, 188–189t
Lips, examination of, 41
Lithotomy position, 235
Liver function tests, 184–186t
Lobar pneumonia, 235
Lobe, defined, 235
Lordosis, 235
Lovenox. *See* heparin
Low-density lipoprotein (LDL), 189t
Lower extremities, fine motor tests for, 49–50
Lower gastrointestinal (LGI) tests
barium enema, defined, 223
purpose of, 198
Lower gastrointestinal (LGI) tests
nursing interventions, 204t
Lumbar puncture (LP, spinal tap), 235
Lumen, defined, 235
Lung compliance, 235
Lung recoil, 235
Lungs. *See also* breath sounds
adults, older, 55–56
compliance and recoil, 235
thorax and lungs, examination of, 42–45, 43t, 44t, 55–56
total lung capacity, 245
Lymph nodes, examination of, 42
Lymphatic, defined, 235
Lymphocytes, 181t

M

Maceration, defined, 235
Magnesium
hypermagnesemia, 231
hypomagnesemia, 232
information about, 215t
normal findings and clinical implications, 192t
Malaise, 235
Males
genitourinary system, review of, for nursing health history, 27
genitourinary system and inguinal area, examination of, 50–51
genitourinary system assessment in older adults, 60
glans penis, 230
prostatectomy, 240
reproductive system, root words for, 169
vasectomy, 247
Malignancy, 235
Malleolus, 235
Malnutrition, 235
Mammography, 235
Manganese, 218t
Mastectomy, 235
Masticate, defined, 236
Mean corpuscular hemoglobin (MCH), 180t
Mean corpuscular hemoglobin concentration (MCHC), 180t
Mean corpuscular volume (MCV), 180t
Measles. *See* rubeola (measles)
Measurement conversions and equivalents, 176–177
Meatus, defined, 236
Medial, defined, 236
Medical asepsis, 236
Medications
dosage calculation, 129–135
nurses' responsibilities, 126–127
older adults, special care for, 127, 129
past history, 23
rights for accurate administration, 125–126
Medications
common abbreviations, 128t
subcutaneous injections, 137f, 142t
intradermal injections, 136f, 142t
intramuscular injections, 138–140f, 141f, 142t
Melanin, 236
Melanotic freckles, 52
Meniscus, defined, 236
Mental health disorders, in family history, 23
Mental status, for general survey, 37–38
Metabolism, 236
Metacarpal, defined, 236
Metric system, 176–177
Microorganisms in urine, 98
Micturate (urinate, void), 236, 248
Midclavicular line, 236

Midsternal line, 236
Minerals
major minerals, 98, 190–192t, 215–216t, 231, 232
trace minerals, 217–219t
Miosis, 239
MMR (measles, mumps, rubella) vaccine, 236
Molybdenum, 218t
Monocytes, 182t
Mons pubis (mons veneris), 236
Montgomery straps, 236
Morbidity, 236
Motor function, 49–50
Mouth
examination of older adults, 54–55
floor of, examination of, 41
physical health examination, 41
review of, for nursing health history, 26
Mucolytic, defined, 239
Mucous membrane, defined, 236
Mucus, 236
Mumps
droplet precautions, 158
MMR vaccine, 236
past history, 23
Murmur (cardiac), 236
Muscles, examination of, 48
Musculoskeletal system
older adults, examination of, 58
physical health examination, 48–49
review of, for nursing health history, 27
Mydriatic, 236
Myelogram
defined, 236
nursing interventions, 210t
Myocardial infarction, 236
Myocardium, 236
Myoglobin level, 187t

N
Nails
older adults, examination of, 52
physical health examination, 38
review of, for nursing health history, 26
NANDA-approved nursing diagnoses, 62–68
Narcotic antagonist, 236
Narrative documentation format, 148–149
Nasogastric tubes
defined, 236
inserting, 92–93
removing, 93
Nasopharyngeal suctioning, 90–91
Nasopharynx, 236
Nausea, 236
Nebulizer, defined, 236
Neck
physical health examination, 42
review of, for nursing health history, 26
Necrosis, 236
Negative nitrogen balance, 236
Neoplasm, 236
Nephritis, 237
Nephron, 237
Nephrosis, 237
Nerve block, 237
Nervous system, root words for, 169
Neurologic, defined, 237
Neurologic system
older adults, examination of, 58–60
physical health examination, 49–50
review of, for nursing health history, 27
Neutrophils, 181t
Niacin, 213t
Nitrite in urine, 98
Nocturia (nycturia), 237
Nocturnal enuresis, 237
Non-English-speaking clients, communication with, 10
Nonproductive cough, 90, 237
Normal breath sounds, 43t
Normal saline, 237
Nose
older adults, examination of, 54
physical health examination, 41
review of, for nursing health history, 26
Nosocomial, defined, 237
Nurses' responsibilities for medication administration, 126–127
Nursing diagnoses
diagnostic statements, formulating, 61–62
NANDA-approved nursing diagnoses, 62–68
Nursing health history
biographic data, 22
chief complaint or reason for visit, 22
family history of illness, 23
health care patterns, 25
history of present illness, 22–23
lifestyle, 24
past history, 23
psychological data, 25

review of systems, 25–27
social data, 24–25
Nursing process, components of, 2–3
Nycturia (nocturia), 237

O

Obesity
defined, 240
family history, 23
Objective data, 237
Observation of respiratory function, 88
Obstructions in urinary system, 98
Obturator, 237
Ointment, 237
Olfactory, defined, 237
Oliguria, 237
Operative (intraoperative) period, 233, 237
Ophthalmoscope, 237
Opportunistic pathogen, 237
Oral medications, rounding numbers for, 130–131
Orientation, defined, 237
Orifice, 237
Oropharyngeal suctioning, 90–91
Oropharynx
defined, 237
physical health examination, 42
Orthopnea, 89, 240
Orthostatic hypotension, 237
Osteoarthritis (arthritis), 23, 237
Osteoporosis
adults, older, 55, 58
defined, 237
Ostomy, defined, 237
Otoscope, 237
Outward rotation, 237
Ova and parasite (O&P) test for stool, 198
Overweight, defined, 237
Oxygen, partial pressure of, 237, 238
Oxygen saturation
procedure for assessment, 34–35
Oxygen saturation
normal findings and clinical implications, 193t

P

Packing, 237
$PaCO_2$, 238
Pain
cognitive-behavioral modalities, 85–86
fecal elimination, 101
older adults, special care for, 87
overview of, 83–85
patient-controlled analgesia pump, 87
postoperative period, 117
urinary elimination, 97
Palate
defined, 238
physical health examination, 41
Palliative, defined, 238
Pallor, 238
Palpation
abdomen, 47
bladder, 47
defined, 238
examination method, 28
Pandemic, defined, 238
Pantothenic acid, 214t
PaO_2, 238
Papule, 238
Paracentesis, 238
Paradoxical breathing, 238
Paralysis, 238
Paraplegia, 238
Parasites, 238
Parenchyma, 238
Parenteral defined, 238
Parenteral medications, 131. *See also* injections
Paresis, 238
Paresthesia, 238
Paronychia, 238
Parotitis (parotiditis), 238
PASS (Pull out safety pin, Aim the hose, Squeeze the handle, Sweep the hose) use of fire extinguishers, 76
Passive exercise, 238
Past history, in nursing health history, 23
Paste, 238
Patent, defined, 238
Pathogen, 238
Patient-controlled analgesia pumps, 87
PCO_2, 238
Peak plasma level (of drug), 238
Pediatric clients, dosage calculation for, 131
Pediculosis, 238
Penetrating wound, 238
Penrose drain, 238
Percussion
abdomen, 47
chest, 88
defined, 238
dullness, 227
examination method, 28–29
flatness, 229

Percutaneous electric stimulation, 238
Percutaneous transhepatic cholangiography, 207t
Perfusion
defined, 238
peripheral, 46
tissue perfusion, 245
Perineum, 238
Perioperative period, 239
Periorbital, 239
Peripheral, defined, 239
Peripheral pulse, 239
Peripheral vascular system
older adults, examination of, 56–57
physical health examination, 45–46
Peristalsis, 239
Peristomal, defined, 239
Peritoneal cavity, 239
Peritoneum, 239
Peritonitis, 239
Perspiration, 239
Pertussis, 158
Petechiae, 239
PH
arterial blood, 193t
defined, 239
urine, 97, 195t
Phalanx, defined, 239
Phantom pain, 239
Phlebitis, 239
Phlebotomy, 239
Phosphorus (phosphate)
information about, 215t
normal findings and clinical implications, 192t
Photosensitive, 239
Physical health examination
abdomen, 47, 48f, 57–58
breasts and axillae, 46–47, 57
cardiovascular and peripheral vascular system, 45–46, 46f, 56–57
female genitals and inguinal lymph nodes, 50, 60
general survey, 37–38
head, 39–42, 53–55
integumentary system, 38, 51–52
male genitals and inguinal area, 50–51, 60
musculoskeletal system, 48–49, 58
neurologic system, 49–50, 58–60
nose and sinuses, 54
older adults, special considerations for, 51–60
preparing the client, 36–37
rectum and anus, 51
Physical health examination
thorax and lungs, 42–45, 43t, 44t, 55–56
Pitch, defined, 239
Pitting edema, 239
Planning, as nursing process component, 2–3
Planning and implementation
clinical guidelines
clients with pain, individualizing care for, 83–87
fecal elimination, 100–103
fluid and electrolyte balance, 77–83
healing wounds, 114–115
postoperative period, 116–118
respiratory function, 87–91
tube feedings, 91–95
urinary elimination, 96–100
medications
dosage calculation, 129–135
nurses' responsibilities, 126–127
older adults, special care for, 127, 129
rights for accurate administration, 125–126
safety guidelines
body mechanics, 71–72
falls, preventing in health care agencies, 73–74
fire, steps to follow with, 75–76
home hazard appraisal, 74–75
importance of, 70–71
safe client handling and movement, 72–73
teaching and learning guidelines, 119–124
Planning and implementation
clinical guidelines
pressure areas, 103–113, 105f, 108–109f, 111–113t
medications
common abbreviations, 128t
subcutaneous injections, 137f, 142t
intradermal injections, 136f, 142t
intramuscular injections, 138–140f, 141f, 142t
Plantar flexion, 239
Plasma, 239
Platelet count, 183t
Pleural rub (friction rub), 44t, 229, 239
Pneumonia
defined, 239
postoperative period, 117
Pneumothorax, 230, 239

PO_2, 239
Polydipsia, 239
Polyneuritis, 239
Polyurethane foam dressings, 113t
Polyuria (diuresis), 227, 239
Popliteal, defined, 239
Port, defined, 239
Position sensation, 50
Posterior, defined, 239
Posterior thorax, examination of, 42–43, 43t, 44t
Postexposure prophylaxis
  hepatitis B virus, 162
  hepatitis C virus, 162
  human immunodeficiency virus (HIV), 161–162
Postoperative cholangiography, 207t
Postoperative (postsurgical) period
  client assessment, 116–117
  complications, signs of, 117–118
  defined, 239
  gastrointestinal suction, 118
  irrigations, 118
Postural drainage, 239
Potassium
  blood levels, and urinary elimination, 98
  hyperkalemia, 231
  hypokalemia, 232
Potassium
  information about, 216t
  normal findings and clinical implications, 190t
Precordium, 239
Prefixes, 170–174
Premature ventricular contractions, 56
Preoperative period, 240
Prepuce. *See* foreskin
Presbycusis, 54
Presbyopia, 53
Pressure areas
  client assessment, 103–106, 105f
  older adults, special care for, 110
  pressure ulcers, preventing, 106–107, 108–109f
  pressure ulcers, treating, 107
  pressure ulcers, wound dressings for, 111–113t
Pressure ulcers
  classification of, 104, 106
  preventing, 106–107, 108–109f
  treating, 107
Primary intention healing (primary union), 240
Problem, in diagnostic statements, 61, 62
Proctoscopy
  defined, 240
Proctoscopy
  nursing interventions, 202t
Prodromal period, 240
Productive cough, 90
Prognosis, 240
Pronation, 240
Prone position, 240
Prophylaxis
  defined, 240
  postexposure, 161–162
Prostatectomy, 240
Prosthesis, 240
Protein in urine
  proteinuria, defined, 240
  urinary elimination, 98
Protein in urine
  normal findings and clinical implications, 195t
Prothrombin time, 186t
Protocol, defined, 240
Proximal, defined, 240
Pruritus, 240
Psychological data, for nursing health history, 25
Ptosis, 240
Pulmonary embolus
  defined, 240
  postoperative period, 117
Pulmonary function tests, 89
Pulse
  defined, 240
  fluid and electrolyte balance, 78
  postoperative period, 116
  procedure for taking, 31
  sites for, 32f
  variations by age, 33
Pulse deficit, 240
Pulse oximetry, 89
Pulse pressure, 240
Pulse rate, defined, 240
Pulse rhythm, 240
Pulse volume, 240
Puncture (stab) wound, 240
Purulent, defined, 240
Pus, 240
Pustule, 240
Putrid, defined, 240
Pyelogram, 240
Pyrexia, 240
Pyridoxine (vitamin B_6), 213t
Pyuria, 241

Q

Quality (of sound), 241

R
RACE (Rescue, Activate, Confine, Extinguish) fire protocol, 75
Radial pulse, 241
Radiating pain, 241
Radiographic (radiologic) tests
  common diagnostic, purpose of, 198
  retrograde pyelogram, 241
  roentgenogram, defined, 242
  tomography, 245
  x-rays, defined, 248
Radiographic (radiologic) tests
  angiography, 209t, 222
  gallbladder and bile ducts, 205–207t, 224, 234
  GI studies, 198, 203–204t, 223
  IV pyelography or urography, 208t, 234
  myelography, 210t, 236
Rales (crackles), defined, 225. *See also* crackles (rales)
Range of motion (ROM), 241
Ratio and proportion method of dosage calculation, 132
RBC. *See* red blood cells (RBCs)
Reason for visit, for nursing health history, 22
Rebound phenomenon (thermal), 241
Reconstitution, defined, 241
Rectum, examination of, 51
Rectus femoris site for intramuscular injections, 139f
Red blood cells (RBCs)
  erythrocyte, defined, 228
  RBC count, 179t
  RBC indices, 180t
Referred pain, 241
Reflex, defined, 241
Reflux, defined, 241
Regeneration, 241
Regurgitation, 241
Rehabilitation, 241
Relaxation response, for pain, 85
Renal, defined, 241
Renal dialysis, 241
Renal pelvis, 241
Repatterning unhelpful thinking, 85–86
Reproductive system, 169. *See also* females; males
Residual urine, 241
Residual volume (air), 241
Resonance, 241
Respiration
  defined, 241
  fluid and electrolyte balance, 78
  postoperative period, 116
  procedure for taking, 33
  variations by age, 33
Respiratory acidosis (hypercapnia), 231, 241
Respiratory arrest, 241
Respiratory function. *See also* breath sounds; lungs
  breathing patterns, breath sounds, and chest movements, abnormal, 89–90
  chest auscultation, 89
  chest palpation, 88
  chest percussion, 88
  client assessment, 87–88
  laboratory tests, 89
  observation of, 88
  older adults, special care for, 91
  oropharyngeal and nasopharyngeal suctioning, 90–91
Respiratory system
  review of, for nursing health history, 26
  root words, 169
Resuscitate, 241
Retching, defined, 241
Retention (urinary), 241
Retention enemas, 103
Retinol (vitamin A), 211t
Retrograde pyelogram, 241
Retroperitoneal, defined, 241
Reverse isolation (barrier technique), 242
Reverse Trendelenburg's position, 242
Review of systems, for nursing health history, 25–27
Rh factor, 242
Rheumatic fever, 23
Rhinitis, 242
Rhonchi (gurgles)
  abnormal breath sound, 90
  defined, 242
  described, cause, and location, 44t
Riboflavin (vitamin B_2), 213t
Right circumstances for delegation, 4
Right direction and communication for delegation, 4
Right person for delegation, 4
Right supervision and evaluation for delegation, 4
Right task for delegation, 4
"Rights" for accurate medication administration, 125–126
"Rights" of delegation, 4
Rinne test, 40

Roentgenogram, defined, 242. *See also* radiographic (radiologic) tests
ROM (range of motion), 242
Romberg's test, 49
Root words
  body systems, 168–169
  regions of the body, 169–170
  tissues, 170
Rotation, defined, 242
Rounding numbers
  IV infusion, 131
  oral medications, 130–131
  parenteral medications, 131
  rounding down, 131
Rubella (German measles)
  droplet precautions, 158
  MMR vaccine, 236
  past history, 23
Rubeola (measles)
  airborne precautions, 158
  MMR vaccine, 236
  past history, 23

S

Safety guidelines
  body mechanics, 71–72
  falls, preventing in health care agencies, 73–74
  fire, steps to follow with, 75–76
  home hazard appraisal, 74–75
  importance of, 70–71
  safe client handling and movement, 72–73
Salem sump tube, 242
Sanguineous, defined, 242
Sanguineous exudate, 242
Saphenous vein, 242
SBAR (Situation, Background, Assessment, Recommendations) communication guidelines, 15–17
Scans, medical, purpose of, 198
Scar tissue (cicatrix), 224, 242
Scarlet fever, 23
Sclerosis, defined, 242
Scoliosis, 242
Sebaceous gland, 242
Seborrheic dermatitis, 242
Seborrheic keratosis, 52
Secondary intention healing, 242
Secretion, defined, 242
Sedative, 242
Selenium, 219t
Semi-Fowler's position, 242
Senile lentigines, 52
Sensitivity, defined, 242
Sensory function, examination of, 50
Septic, defined, 242
Serosanguineous, defined, 243
Serous exudate, 243
Serum. *See* blood (serum)
Serum osmolality, 192t
Shock, defined, 243
Sickle cell, 243
Side effect, defined, 243
Sigmoidoscopy
  defined, 243
  nursing interventions, 202t
Signs and symptoms, in diagnostic statements, 61, 62
Sinuses
  older adults, examination of, 54
  physical health examination, 41
Sitz bath (hip bath), 243
Skeletal system, 169. *See also* musculoskeletal system
Skin. *See also* wounds
  color and temperature
    postoperative period, 116
    pressure areas, 106
  integument, defined, 233
  older adults, examination of, 51–52
  palpation of pressure areas, 106
  physical health examination, 38
Skull, examination of, 39
Sleep apnea, 243
Smear, defined, 243
SOAP (Subjective, Objective, Assessment, Planning) documentation format, 149, 150–151f
SOAPIE (Subjective, Objective, Assessment, Planning, Implementation, Evaluation) documentation format, 149, 150–151
SOAPIER (Subjective, Objective, Assessment, Planning, Implementation, Evaluation, Revision) documentation format, 149, 150–151f
Social data, for nursing health history, 24–25
Sodium
  blood levels, and urinary elimination, 98
  hypernatremia, 231
  hyponatremia, 232
  information about, 216t
  normal findings and clinical implications, 190t
Spasm, defined, 243

Specific gravity
defined, 243
urine
fluid and electrolyte balance, 79
urinary elimination, 97
Specific gravity
urine
normal values and possible etiologies, 195t
Speculum, 243
Sphincter, defined, 243
Sphygmomanometer, 243
Spinal tap (lumbar puncture), 235
Spiritual interventions for pain, 86
Spirometry, 243
Splint, 243
Sprain, 243
Sputum
defined, 243
tests on, 89, 197
Stab (puncture) wound, 240
Stairway hazards, 74
Standard precautions, guidelines for, 156–157
Staphylococcus aureus, 159
Stasis, defined, 243
Stenosis, defined, 243
Sterile, defined, 243
Sterile technique. *See* surgical asepsis
Sterilization, defined, 243
Stertor, 90, 243
Stethoscope, 243
Stoma, defined, 243
Stool (feces). *See also* fecal elimination
color and consistency, 101
defined, 228, 243
tests on, 198
Stopcock, defined, 243
Strain (of a muscle), 243
Streptococcal infections, past history of, 23
Stridor, 89, 235, 244
Stroke volume, 244
Stupor, 244
Stylet, 244
Subcostal, defined, 244
Subcutaneous (hypodermic), defined, 244
Subcutaneous injections
sites for, 137f
Subcutaneous injections
sites, needles, syringes, mounts, angles, 142t
Subjective data, 244
Sublingual, defined, 244
Suborbital, defined, 244
Subscapular, defined, 244
Substernal retractions, 90, 244
Suffixes, 174–175
Sulfur, 216t
Supination, 244
Supine position, 244
Suppository, 244
Supraclavicular retractions, 244
Suprapubic, defined, 244
Suprasternal retractions, 90, 244
Surfactant, 244
Surgical asepsis, 244
Sustained maximal inspiration [SMI] device (incentive spirometer), 233
Suture, defined, 244
Symptoms (covert data). *See* subjective data
Syncope, 244
Syndrome, defined, 244
Synovial joint, 244
Syphilis, 244
Syringe, defined, 244
Systemic, defined, 244
Systole, 245
Systolic pressure, 245

T

Tablet, 245
Tachycardia, 245
Tachypnea, 89, 245
Tactile (vocal) fremitus, 245
TB. *See* tuberculosis (TB)
T-binder, 245
Td (tetanus and diphtheria toxoids), 245
Teaching and learning
guidelines for, 120–122
older adults, special care for, 123–124
settings, for, 119–120
teaching process, steps in, 119
Teeth, examination of, 41
Telangiectasias, 52
Telephone orders, guidelines for, 19–20
Temperature. *See* body temperature
Temporal pulse, 245
Tenesmus, 245
TENS (transcutaneous electrical nerve stimulation), 246
Terminology
prefixes, 170–174
root words, 168–170
suffixes, 174–175
Tetany, 245

Therapeutic communication techniques, 7
Therapy, defined, 245
Thiamin (vitamin B_1), 212t
Thorax
  older adults, examination of, 55
Thorax
  physical health examination, 42–45, 43t, 44t
Three-part diagnostic statements, 61–62
Throat, review of, for nursing health history, 26
Thrombocytopenia, 245
Thrombophlebitis
  defined, 245
  postoperative period, 117
Thrombosis, defined, 245
Thrombus
  defined, 245
  postoperative period, 117
Thyroid gland, examination of, 42
Tic, defined, 245
Tidal volume, 245
Tinnitus, 245
Tissue perfusion, 245
Tocopherol (vitamin E), 212t
Tomography, 245
Tongue, examination of, 41
Tonicity, defined, 245
Tonsils, examination of, 42
Tonus, defined, 245
Topical, defined, 245
Tortuous, defined, 245
Total lung capacity, 245
Total parenteral nutrition (intravenous hyperalimentation), 245
Tourniquet, 246
Toxemia, 246
Toxic substances in the home, 75
Toxin, defined, 246
Trace minerals, 217–219t
Trachea, examination of, 42
Tracheal tug, 246
Tracheostomy, 246
Traction, defined, 246
Trademark (brand name), 246
Transcutaneous electrical nerve stimulation (TENS), 246
Transfusion, defined, 246
Transmission-based precautions
  airborne precautions, 158
  contact precautions, 159
  droplet precautions, 158
  standard precautions, with, 157–158
Transparent film dressings, 111t
Trapeze bar, 246
Trauma, defined, 246
Tremor, defined, 246
Trendelenburg's position, 246
Triglyceride level, 189t
Trocar, defined, 246
Trochanter, 246
Trochanter roll, 246
Troche, 246
Troponin I level, 187t
Troponin T level, 187t
Tube feedings
  administering, 93–94
  client assessment, 91–92
  gastrostomy or jejunostomy feedings, 94–95
  nasogastric tube, inserting, 92–93
  nasogastric tube, removing, 93
  older adults, special care for, 95
Tuberculosis (TB)
  airborne precautions, 158
  family history, 23
  tuberculin (TB) skin test, 198
Tumor, defined, 246
Tuning fork
  defined, 246
  tests, 40
Turgor, defined, 246
Two-part diagnostic statements, 61
Tympanic membrane, examination of, 40
Tympanites, 118
Tympany, defined, 246

U

UGI test. *See* upper gastrointestinal (UGI) test
Ulcer, defined, 246
Ultrasound, 246
Unconscious, defined, 246
Unilateral, defined, 246
Unit dose system (of drugs), 246
Universal donor, 246
Universal recipient, 247
Unlicensed assistive personnel
  principles for delegation to, 5–6
Unlicensed assistive personnel
  tasks that may and may not be delegated to, 5t
Unsterile, defined, 247
Upper extremities, fine motor tests for, 49
Upper gastrointestinal (UGI) test
  purpose of, 198
Upper gastrointestinal (UGI) test
  nursing interventions, 203t

Urea, 247
Ureterostomy, 247
Urethritis, 247
Urgency (urinary), 247
Uric acid, in urine, 195t
Urinal, 247
Urinalysis
  defined, 247
  normal findings and clinical implications, 194–195t
  purpose of, 198
  urinary elimination, 97–98
Urinary diversion. *See* urostomy
Urinary elimination
  anuria, 222
  client assessment, 96–98
  diuresis (polyuria), 227, 239
  factors influencing, 97
  history, 96
  laboratory tests and examinations, 97–98
  older adults, special care for, 99–100
  oliguria, 237
  pain, 97
  postoperative period, 117
  retention catheter, removing, 99
  urinary catheterization, 98
  urine, volume and characteristics of, 96–97
  void (micturate, urinate), defined, 236, 248
Urinary infection
  bacteriuria, 222
  postoperative period, 118
Urinary system, root words for, 169
Urinate (micturate, void), 236
Urine culture and sensitivity, 198
Urobilinogen
  defined, 247
  urine, in, 98
Urostomy (ureterostomy, urinary diversion), 247
Urticaria, 247
Uvula
  defined, 247
  physical health examination, 41

V

Vaccine, defined, 247
Valsalva maneuver, 247
Varicella, 158
Varicosity, defined, 247
Vasectomy, 247
Vasoconstriction, 247
Vasodilation, 247
Vasopressor, defined, 247
Vasospasm, 247
Vastus lateralis site for intramuscular injections, 138f
Veins, peripheral, examination of, 46
Ventilation, defined, 247
Ventral, defined, 247
Ventricle, defined, 247
Ventrogluteal site for intramuscular injections, 138f
Verbal orders, guidelines for, 19–20
Vertigo, 247
Vesicular sounds
  breath sounds, 43t
  defined, 247
Vial, defined, 247
Vibration, defined, 247
Virulence, defined, 247
Virus, defined, 247
Viscera, 248
Viscosity, defined, 248
Vision
  older adults, examination of, 53
  physical health examination, 39–40
Visual acuity, 40
Visual fields, 39
Vital capacity, 248
Vital (cardinal) signs
  blood pressure, 33–34
  defined, 248
  fecal elimination, 101
  fluid and electrolyte balance, 78
  oxygen saturation, 34–35
  postoperative period, 116
  pulse, 31, 32f, 33
  respirations, 33
  temperature, 30–31
Vitamin A (retinol), 211t
Vitamin B_1 (thiamin), 212t
Vitamin B_2 (riboflavin), 213t
Vitamin B_6 (pyridoxine), 213t
Vitamin B_{12} (cobalamin), 213t
Vitamin C (ascorbic acid), 214t
Vitamin D (calciferol), 211t
Vitamin E (tocopherol), 212t
Vitamin K, 212t
Vitamins
  fat-soluble, 211–212t
  water-soluble, 212–214t
Vitiligo, 52, 253
Vocal (tactile) fremitus, 245
Vocal resonance, 248
Void (micturate, urinate), defined, 236, 248
Volume conversions and equivalents, 177
Vomitus, 248

W
Walker, 248
Walkway hazards, 74
Water-soluble vitamins, 212–214t
WBC. *See* white blood cell (WBC)
Weber's test
  defined, 248
  physical health examination, 40
Weight
  baseline and daily, and fluid and electrolyte balance, 78
  obesity, 23, 237
  overweight, defined, 237
Weight conversions and equivalents, 176–177
Wheal (bleb), 223
Wheeze
  defined, 90, 248
  described, cause, and location, 44t
White blood cell (WBC)
  differential count, 181–182t
  WBC count, normal findings and clinical implications, 181t
Wounds
  abrasion, defined, 221
  closed, 225
  dressings for, 111–113t
  healing
    client assessment, 114
    damp-to-damp dressings, applying, 115
    dry sterile dressing, changing, 114–115
    older adults, special care for, 115
  incision, defined, 233
  lacerate, defined, 234
  postoperative infection, 118
  pressure ulcers, 104, 106–107, 108–109f

X
X-rays, defined, 248
Xyphoid process, 248

Z
Zinc, 219t
Z-track method of intramuscular injections, 141f